AF684166

Copyright © 2022 Allison Tuxbury

The Complete Anti-Inflammatory Cookbook For Diabetes: 125 Nutritionist-Verified Recipes To Provide Rapid Relief & Results for Diabetes, Plus Easy-To-Follow 21-Day Meal Plan With Organic, Nutrient-Rich & Safe Ingredients for Diabetes.

All rights reserved. No part of this guide may be reproduced in any form without permission in writing from the publisher except in the case of brief quotations embodied in critical articles or reviews.

EMPIRE Publishing
20212 Champion Forest Dr. #303
Spring, TX 77379
www.empireghostwriter.com/book-process
@empirepubishing

Legal & Disclaimer
The information contained in this book and its contents is not designed to replace or take the place of any form of medical or professional advice; and is not meant to replace the need for independent medical, financial, legal or other professional advice or services, as may be required.

The content and information in this book has been provided for educational and entertainment purposes only. The content and information contained in this book has been compiled from sources deemed reliable, and it is accurate to the best of the Author's knowledge, information and belief. However, the Author cannot guarantee its accuracy and validity and cannot be held liable for any errors and/or omissions. Further, changes are periodically made to this book as and when needed. Where appropriate and/or necessary, you must consult a professional (including but not limited to your doctor, attorney, financial advisor or such other professional advisor) before using any of the suggested remedies, techniques, or information in this book.

Upon using the contents and information contained in this book, you agree to hold harmless the Author from and against any damages, costs, and expenses, including any legal fees potentially resulting from the application of any of the information provided by this book. This disclaimer applies to any loss, damages or injury caused by the use and application, whether directly or indirectly, of any advice or information presented, whether for breach of contract, tort, negligence, personal injury, criminal intent, or under any other cause of action.

You agree to accept all risks of using the information presented inside this book.

You agree that by continuing to read this book, where appropriate and/or necessary, you shall consult a professional (including but not limited to your doctor, attorney, or financial advisor or such other advisor as needed) before using any of the suggested remedies, techniques, or information in this book.

TABLE OF CONTENTS

TABLE OF CONTENTS

TABLE OF CONTENTS

TABLE OF CONTENTS

TABLE OF CONTENTS

TABLE OF CONTENTS

TABLE OF CONTENTS

TABLE OF CONTENTS

TABLE OF CONTENTS

CHAPTER ONE:
Introduction

INTRODUCTION

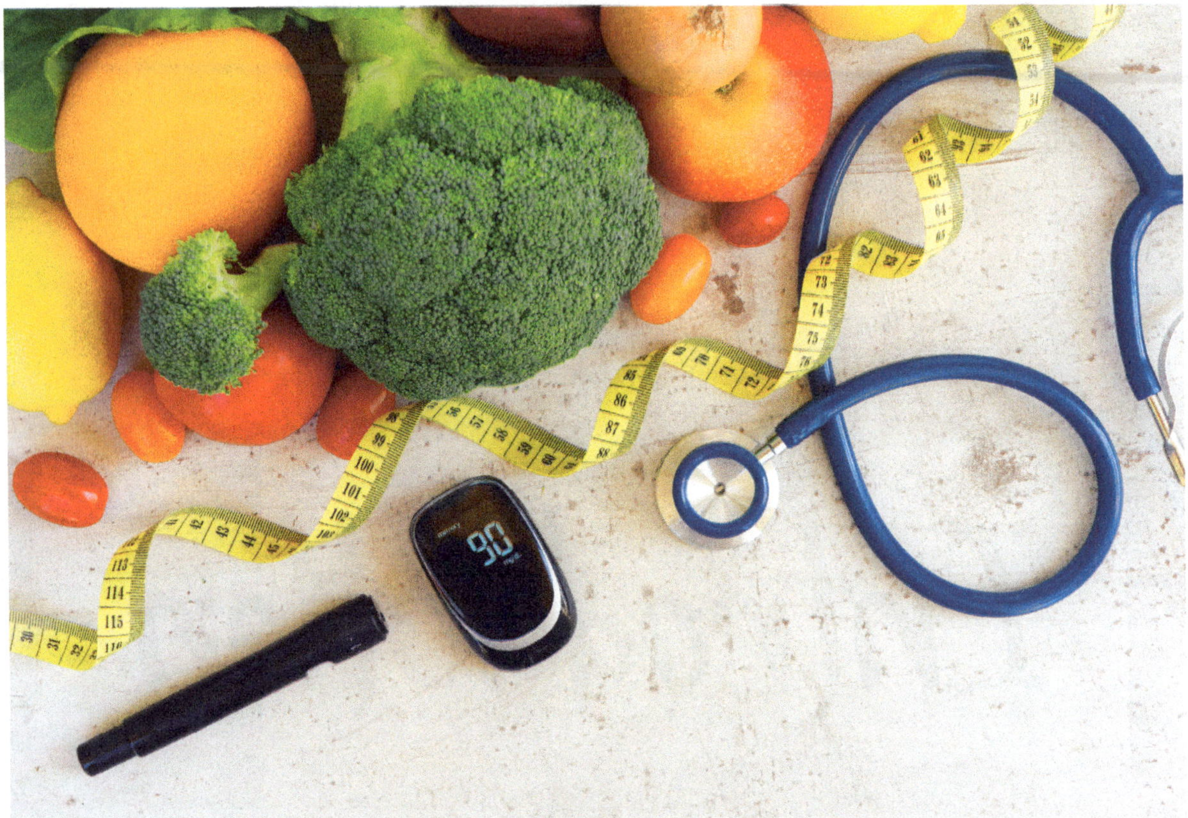

The dreaded diabetes diagnosis. Maybe you've been coping with your condition for a while now, or maybe it's something that has recently been discovered and diagnosed. Either way, it's no fun being told that you have a lifelong condition to manage.

As it is, we are all trying to balance our time, jobs, families, and budgets with enough on our plates. But diabetes doesn't have to damage your life. In fact, it can catapult you into a whole new way of thinking about your health—a new perspective on how the food you eat can support the healthy lifestyle you want to live. And that is what this book is all about.

This cookbook is a tool to help you manage your specific dietary needs to support your life with diabetes, whether you've had it all your life or have just been diagnosed. Gone are the days of diabetes being debilitating or feeling like a depressing prison sentence with no more sweet things to ever grace your taste buds.

Thanks to all the variety in the foods we have available to us today, and all the advances in the medical sciences, there are so many options for how you can effectively manage your diabetes and still enjoy a tasty, nourishing diet that allows you to eat the flavors you love and feel your very best. All the while, you will still be doing your best to avoid any further complications down the road.

So, buckle in and let's delve into what diabetes really is and how it affects your body. This knowledge will teach you how to best support the healthy, happy, and flavorful life you want to live to the fullest!

DIABETES DEBACLE

How did you get here? Well, take comfort in the fact that you aren't alone. Nearly 9.4% of the American population is affected by diabetes.

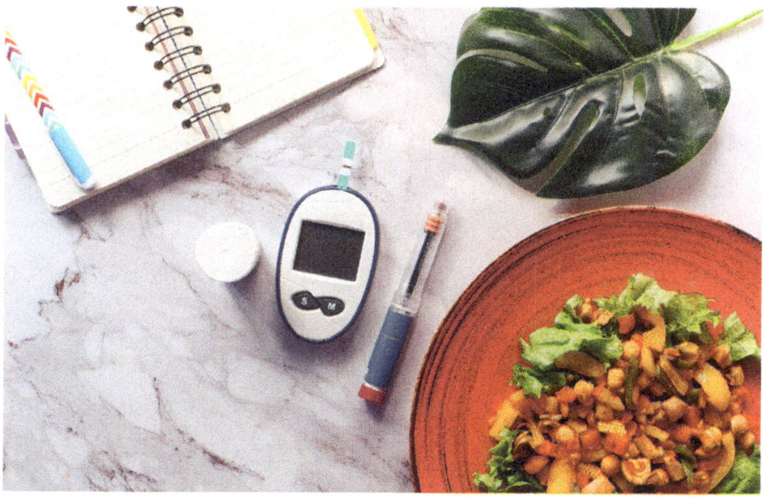

As for how you got your diagnosis, that depends on the type of diabetes you have.

There are two types of diabetes—type 1 and type 2, both of which are a metabolic disease in which high blood sugar levels result from problems in either insulin secretion, or with the body's ability to use the insulin.

Since insulin is the hormone responsible for controlling your body's blood glucose levels, when it isn't functioning as it should, the uptake of glucose into the body's cells is impacted.

With type 1 diabetes, the pancreas cannot produce enough insulin. With type 2, there is instead a resistance to insulin that renders the cells unable to effectively use the insulin that is produced.

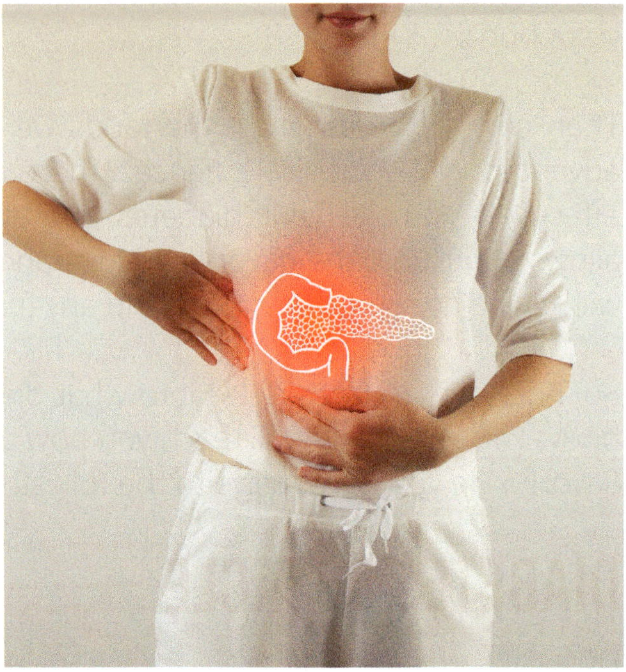

A family history of diabetes can put you at greater risk for type 1 diabetes. However, type 2 diabetes has a wider array of possible causes, ranging from obesity, high blood pressure, elevated cholesterol, and a sedentary lifestyle.

Regardless of which type of diabetes you have, your body's need for a delicate balance of glucose and its reliance on insulin to get the job done are both affected. When you eat, your blood glucose levels rise after a meal. The pancreas releases more insulin into your bloodstream to help glucose be absorbed into the cells and into your bloodstream for your body to use.

Glucose is an essential nutrient that provides your body with energy, so the regulation of glucose levels is critical, even in someone without diabetes. But for people who suffer from diabetes, the glucose levels are off balance and not within normal range. This outcome can lead to a whole host of problems and symptoms, including some pretty severe complications if the disease isn't managed.

NOT AS SWEET AS IT SOUNDS

While diabetes commonly invokes the thought of "too many sweets," there is nothing sweet at all about some of the symptoms this condition can cause. Even in the early stages of the disease, you may find yourself always feeling the urge to pee.

That's because frequent urination is an early sign of diabetes and can quickly lead to dehydration, thereby becoming a repeating cycle before long. Symptoms like fatigue, nausea, vomiting, and frequent infections are also common signs of diabetes.

Sometimes the condition can begin as asymptomatic, so a blood test is necessary to accurately diagnose diabetes in order to measure blood sugar levels. But once you receive your diagnosis, it's time to measure where you're at and get started on a treatment plan you can live with. Educating yourself and using tools such as this cookbook are a great place to start! You want to support your body in the best ways possible so that it can continue to work its hardest to provide you with a healthy, happy, and full life!

Although having diabetes can make you feel a bit defeated at times, there is a definite upside to this condition—you can do a lot to manage it by making some healthy lifestyle changes, including a nourishing diet that is sensitive to your body's special glucose needs and regular exercise to maintain a healthy weight.

Depending on which type of diabetes you have, your medical professional with come up with a treatment plan that is just right for you, usually with a combination of medications, dietary modifications, an active lifestyle, and careful monitoring. So truly, there is no reason to fret—diabetes is one of the most manageable conditions out there that can let you stay in charge of your health!

Ready to get started? Let's talk about which type of diabetes you're dealing with and go from there.

SORRY, BUT YOU'RE JUST NOT MY TYPE

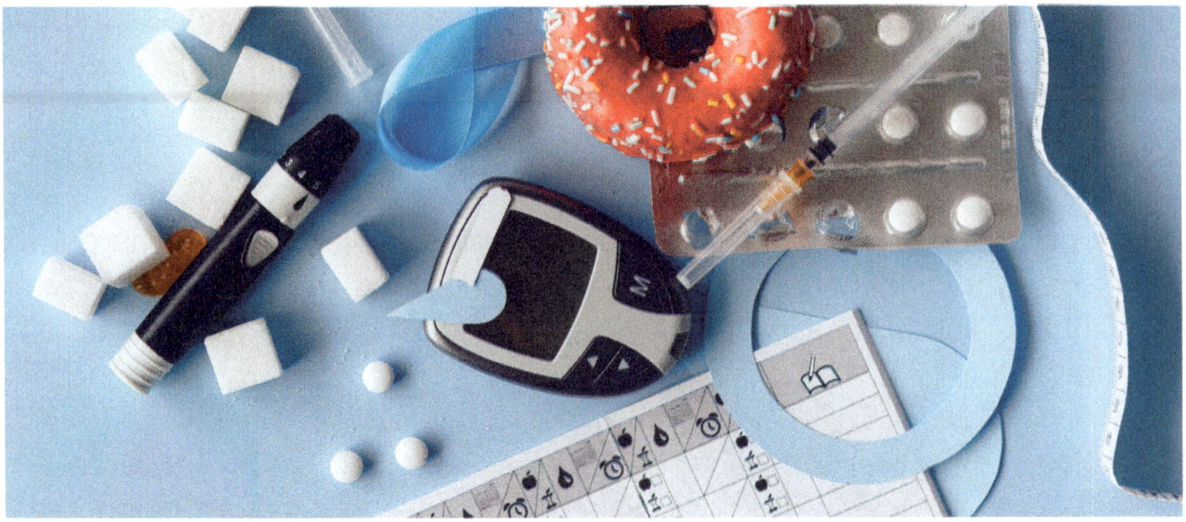

Type 1 and type 2 diabetes function very differently. If you've been diagnosed with type 1 diabetes, you will need to be on insulin medication for the rest of your life to counteract your body's attack on your own immune system. As a result, you'll give your body the insulin it needs in order to function.

If you have type 2 diabetes, then you're in good company, given that this type consists of 90% of all people diagnosed with diabetes. Type 2 diabetes has strong links to poor eating habits and obesity, which means that even if you are already suffering from the condition, making changes to your eating and exercise habits can go a long way in managing your disease and mitigating your symptoms to prevent more serious complications.

Whatever type you have, it will be vital to check your blood sugar levels on a regular regimen, stick to whatever medications prescribed by your doctor, and pay very close attention to your diet, which should support a healthy glycemic load. You may need to modify your exercise routine to keep your body at a healthy weight and see your ophthalmologist regularly "to keep an eye on" diabetic-related complications that may arise.

Diabetes is a condition that frequently involves a whole team of medical professionals, dieticians, and your own commitment to monitoring your health. But instead of seeing your condition as extra work, try to view it as a golden opportunity to take control of your health and educate yourself on ensuring you are living your best and healthiest life possible!

Sure, checking daily blood sugar multiple times a day can be a drag, but just think about how much that action puts you in the driver's seat when dealing with your condition!

If you can keep your glucose levels within normal range before and after eating meals, and collect all the information you can on how your body is functioning in relation to your diet, exercise, medication, and lifestyle modifications, you'll have all the tools you need to manage your diabetes and deal with any symptoms or complications that may arise.

Stay focused on your goal here—to manage your condition, avoid complications, and lead a healthy, happy, and independent life!

CONUNDRUM OF COMPLICATIONS

Yeah, we know—complications suck. But as much as we would all like to not think about all the things that could go wrong, it's important to educate yourself about the potential complications of diabetes so that you can do everything within your power to ensure that you never have to face them.

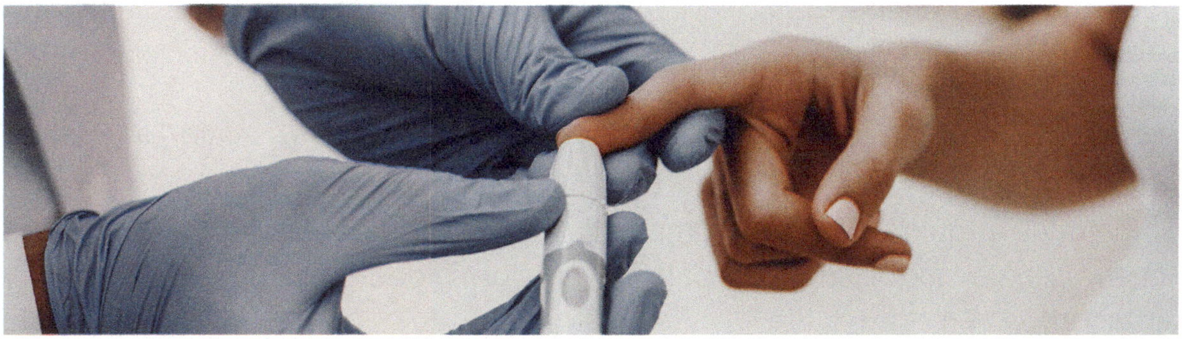

Diabetes can have both acute and chronic complications that can vary depending on—you guessed it—the type of diabetes you have. For people suffering with type 1 diabetes, insulin is vital.

If you have type 1 diabetes, you quite simply cannot survive without an external source of insulin. If you don't get the insulin you need, you could be at risk of a condition called diabetic ketoacidosis, which, without fast medical attention, can lead someone to go into shock or even a coma.

That is because people with type 1 diabetes can develop severely high blood sugar levels, and their lack of insulin can wreak havoc on the process of storing and breaking down fats and proteins in the body, which can cause the release of ketones into the blood.

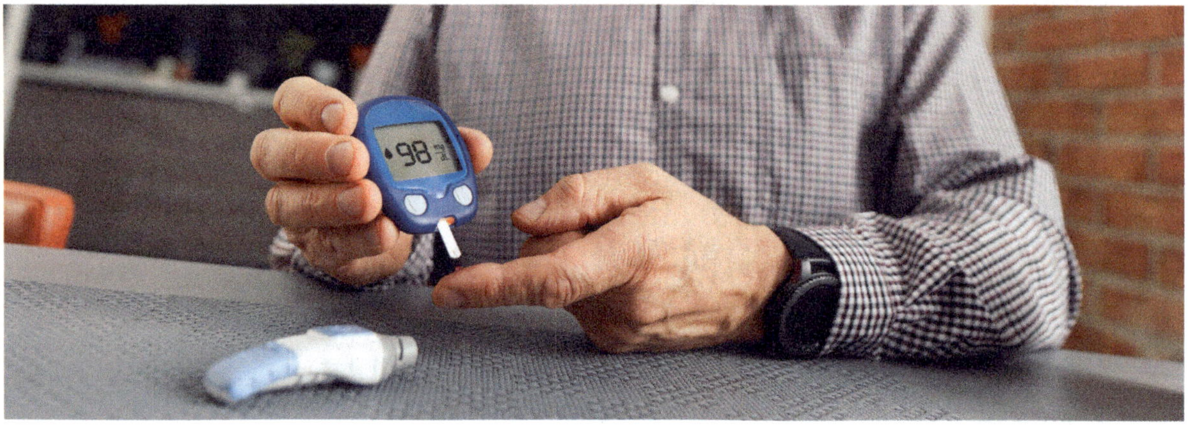

If you are suffering from type 2 diabetes, elevated blood sugar levels or abnormally low blood sugar levels can also lead to a coma condition and seizures.

Regardless of which type of diabetes you have, the goal is to avoid all of these acute complications, which can be life-threatening if not quickly treated. Sometimes, a quick remedy is simply to have a glucose source with you at all times—a quick fix of sugar to balance out low blood sugar in an emergency situation.

But diabetes also has a chronic complication side to its component. Many chronic complications caused by diabetes have to do with blood vessel diseases, which can affect the eyes, kidneys, nerves, and your heart and arteries.

These are all vital components of your body, which is why it's crucial for people with diabetes to maintain optimal cardiovascular health. Keeping good control and management over your condition and monitoring your diabetes vigilantly can stave off common eye complications that can result from poorly managed blood sugar and blood pressure.

Many of the more severe complications of diabetes can be entirely avoided with proper management and monitoring of your condition. Over time, if severe diabetes is left to run wild and isn't properly cared for, the risk of suffering severe complications increases. That's why the best thing you can do for yourself is face your diagnosis head-on and use all the many tools you have at your disposal to build a healthy diet and lifestyle that will support the management of your blood sugar levels.

Your prognosis with diabetes is very closely tied to how well you can keep your condition under control, and that's good news! You have the power to avoid serious complications and live a long and healthy life as long as you take care of yourself and meet the unique needs your body requires.

Remember, your body is not the enemy, and it is working hard to keep you healthy and happy day in and day out. It's your job to ensure that it has all the tools and attention it needs in order to do so!

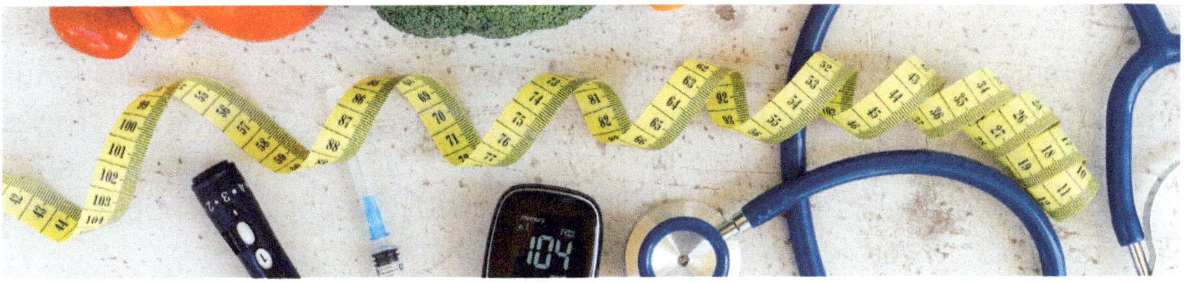

READY TO RUMBLE

You might be aching to to check out the enticing pictures of recipes just a few pages ahead in this book, and that rumbling sound in your stomach is egging you on. But hang on for just a little longer because we've reached the best part! We've talked about your symptoms and the complications you want to avoid, and now it's time to talk about just how to achieve this glorious state of managing your diabetes so that it doesn't manage you!

Don't forget that the entire goal of managing your condition is to keep your glucose levels as close to normal range as safely as possible. For type 1 diabetes, that means insulin, and for type 2 diabetes, that can sometimes mean medications to control elevated blood sugar levels. But for both types of diabetes, the greatest control you have is by implementing a healthy diabetes-sensitive diet and exercise plan.

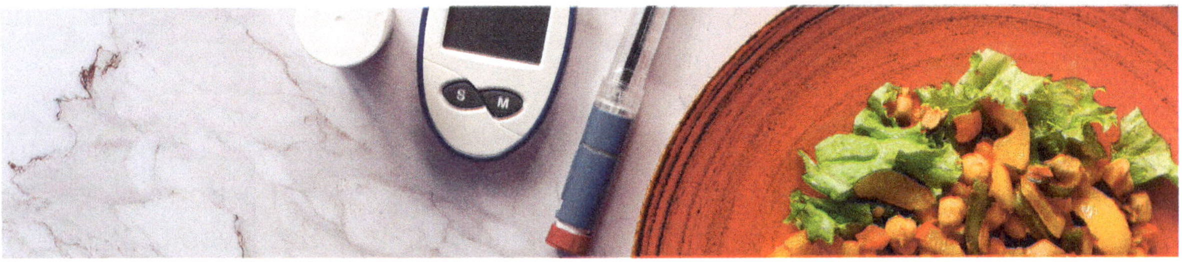

With type 1 diabetes, you'll be monitoring your blood glucose levels throughout the day and balancing your insulin intake with your food and physical exertion. For type 2 diabetes, you'll also be carefully monitoring your diet and exercise, while also possibly adding some medications to control your blood sugar levels from reaching either of the two extremes—too low or too high.

The common thread with both types is that nutrition is key. Sure, nutrition is important for everyone, but for people trying to manage diabetes, it's crucial. Your most single important focus is to control your blood glucose level. Secondly, your goal is to maintain a healthy body weight and support your cardiovascular system.

As with many other health conditions, every person is unique, so there is no one healthy diet that will suit everyone optimally. That is why monitoring and paying careful attention to both your body and your own preferences is so important. You'll need to create an eating plan that fits your individual needs, your schedule and budget, your tastes and habits, and the fluid needs of your body in relation to your glucose levels and symptoms.

You will need to balance your diet along with your exercise habits, insulin, or medications. Sometimes, eating small meals throughout the day can help keep your levels more stable, and with some pre-planning and portion control, you can eat pretty much whatever you want without having to completely eliminate certain foods from your diet. You'll become an expert in how to carefully raise and lower your blood sugar levels and keep things under control.

Does all this sound like a lot of work? That's why we're here to help you out with this amazing cookbook! We've taken all the guesswork out of meal planning and done the research for you.

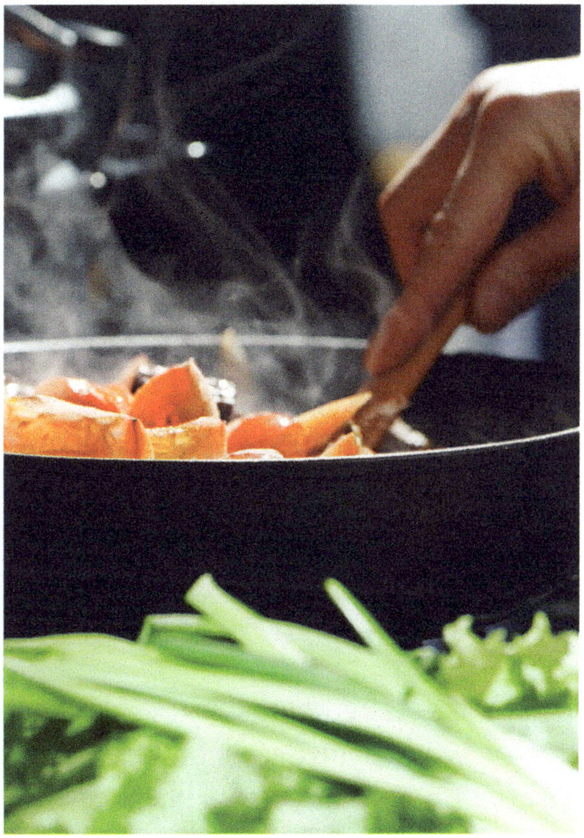

We've carefully considered the nutritional needs of someone with diabetes, the importance of glycemic load and portion sizes, and the nutrient-dense foods that will support your body. We've even included ingredients suspected to help stabilize blood glucose levels, like garlic, cinnamon, and magnesium. And we've compiled it all into one book that is a veritable wonderland of enjoyable recipes for you to try.

You're already dealing with diabetes, so there's no reason for you to also have to worry about tedious meal prep, time-consuming trips to the grocery store, or taste-depriving dishes that leave you feeling unsatisfied.

This cookbook is filled with valuable tips and tricks and loads of healthy, delectable recipes that will help you manage your disease. You won't feel like you are missing out on anything, and you won't be spending precious time or valuable resources trying to make delicious meals to sustain your health.

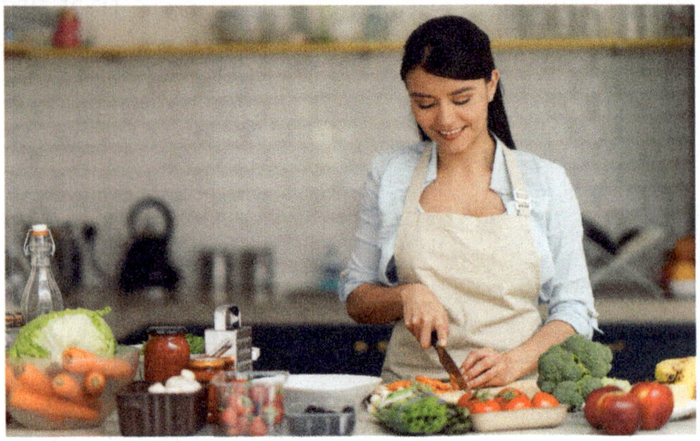

Instead, all you need to do is flip through the pages of this book, pick out the recipes you want to try, make any modifications in line with your tastes, and get started! Every dish has been carefully thought out with your diabetic condition in mind to best nourish your body and support its peak functioning.

The meals inside these pages are carefully balanced, based on research, and are both easy to follow and easy to adjust. Of course, always follow the advice of your medical professional and dietician. Then, sit back and enjoy these recipes that will delight all your senses.

Diabetes doesn't mean that a life of restrictions, and it certainly doesn't mean that you can't easily prepare and enjoy delicious foods with your family and friends. In fact, your condition gives you all the more reason to explore new taste combinations and educate yourself on keeping your body in perfectly balanced health.

You've likely already taken the few first steps in managing your condition—from doctor visits to insulin shots to medication treatment plans. Now, you're ready for the fun part—this cookbook!

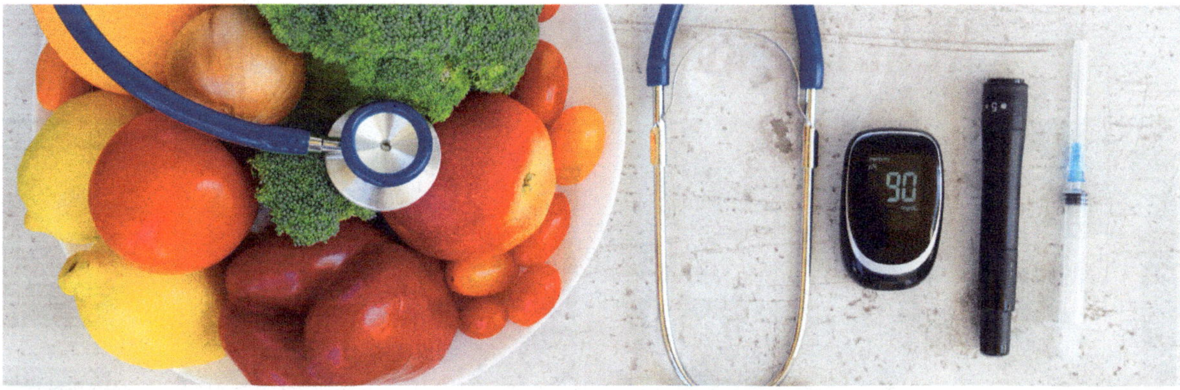

You've got a great tool in your hands, and a partner on your nutritional journey to meet the needs of your condition. And just because this cookbook is geared toward your needs doesn't mean that it won't still be a hit with those around you who enjoy good meals as well!

Every recipe has been tried and tested, and our tastebuds approve! We've gone the extra mile to ensure that the dishes in this book are unique and interesting plus pleasing to look at, taste, and even smell. After all, part of your journey with managing your diabetes is to ensure that you live a full life without sacrificing the things you enjoy, and for many people, that means food!

So, sit back and get ready to see some mouth-watering new meals to create on the pages ahead because you've earned it. You've learned about diabetes and the importance of keeping your levels in check while monitoring your condition meticulously—now's the time to start taking your very first bite out of the rest of your life with your diabetes under tight control.

As you will soon see, just because your condition will be regulated and kept under strict watch, your meals will continue to be as creative as anyone else with or without diabetes. Get excited, stay on top of your glucose levels with careful monitoring, and dig into a whole new world of exquisitely crafted meals!

You can thank us later, after you've enjoyed your meal.

HEALTHY RECIPES FOR DIABETES

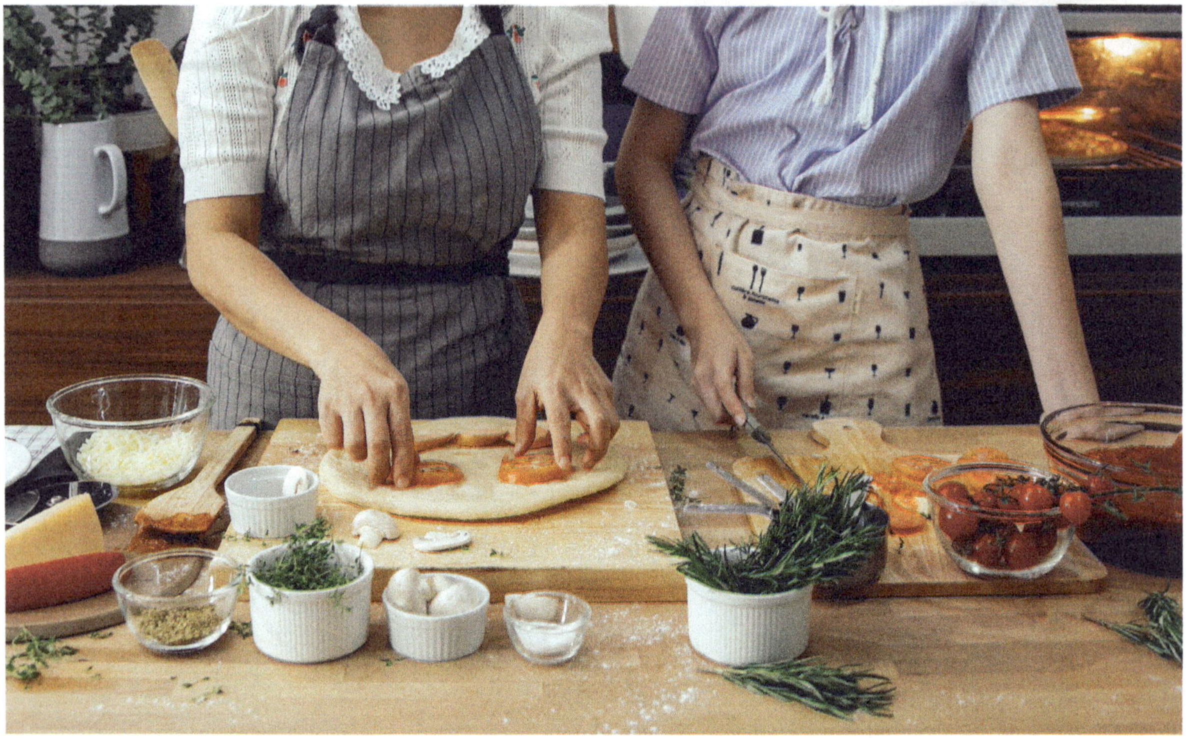

Since you have diabetes, it's important to eat a balanced and healthy diet. That doesn't mean that your food has to be boring! This book is full of delicious recipes for every meal of the day that are good for you AND taste great.

Inside, you'll find 25 snacks, 25 breakfasts, 25 lunches, 25 dinners, and 25 desserts that are all sugar-free, low-fat, and sodium-free. Plus, they're all neutral or beneficial for diabetes! So go ahead and enjoy yourself without feeling guilty or worrying about your health.

Bon appetit!

CHAPTER TWO:

Snacks

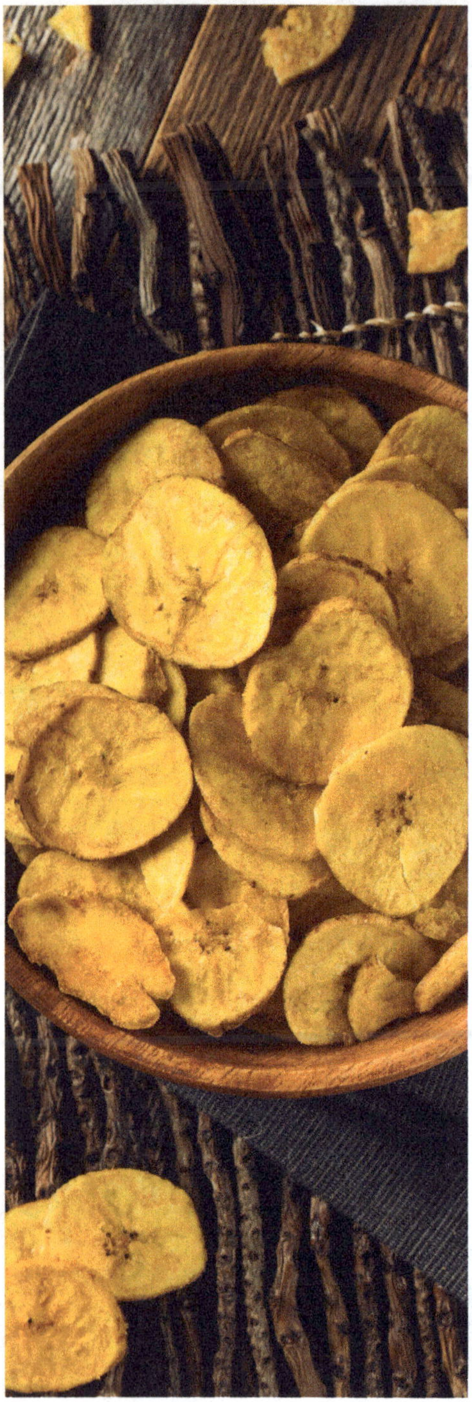

AIR FRYER PLANTAIN CHIPS

Ingredients:

- 2 large green plantains, sliced into thin chips
- 1 tablespoon olive oil
- Salt (optional) to taste

Instructions:

1. Preheat air fryer to 375 degrees F.
2. In a large bowl, toss together plantain chips and olive oil. Season with salt (optional) to taste.
3. Spread in an even layer in the basket of the air fryer and cook for 10 minutes, or until chips are golden brown and crispy. Serve immediately!

Serving Size: 1/2 cup
Calories: 120

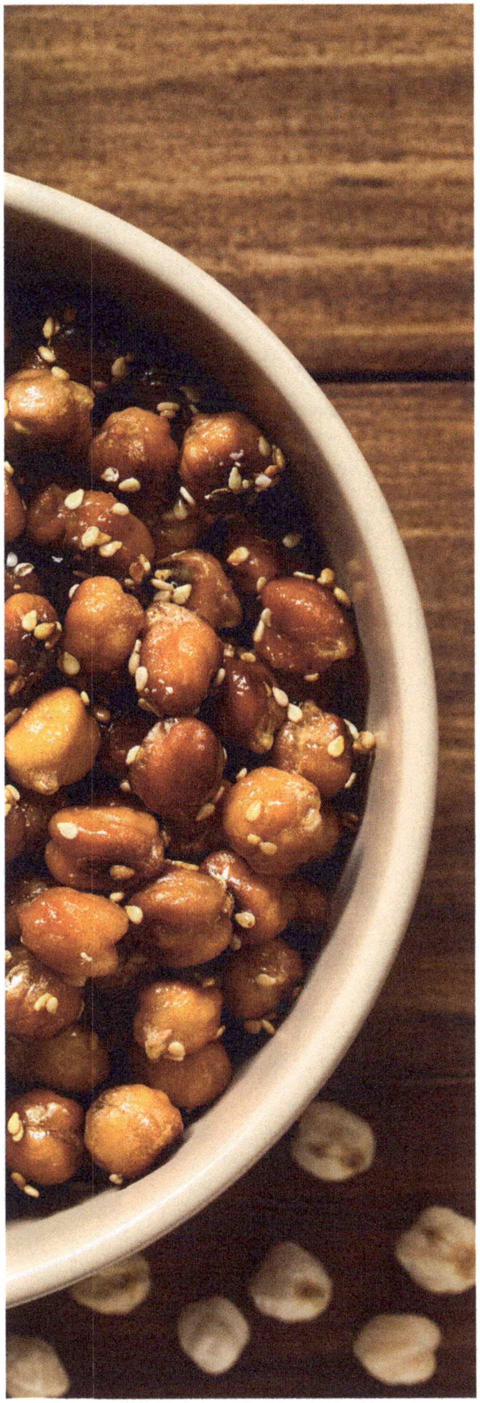

SPICY ROASTED CHICKPEAS

Ingredients:

- 1 (15-ounce) can chickpeas, drained and rinsed
- 1 tablespoon olive oil
- 1 teaspoon chili powder
- 1/2 teaspoon ground cumin
- Salt (optional) and black pepper (optional) to taste

Instructions:

1. Preheat oven to 375 degrees F.
2. In a large bowl, toss together chickpeas, olive oil, chili powder, and cumin. Season with salt and black pepper (optional) to taste.
3. Spread in an even layer on a baking sheet and roast for 15-20 minutes, or until chickpeas are crispy. Serve immediately!

Serving Size: 1/2 cup
Calories: 130

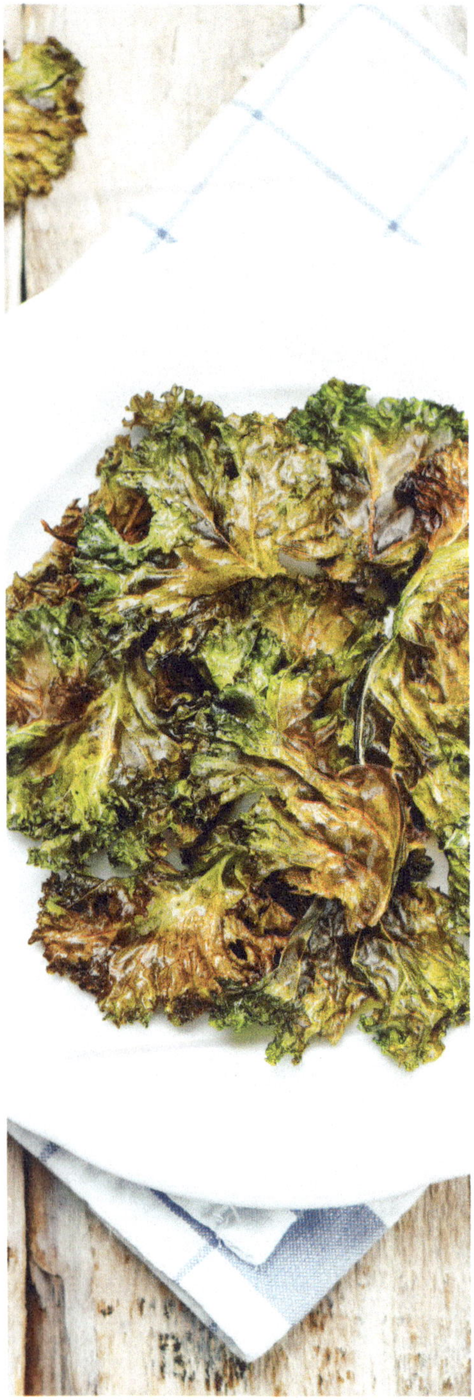

CHEESY KALE CHIPS

Ingredients:

- 1 bunch kale, washed and dried
- 1 tablespoon olive oil
- Salt (optional) and black pepper (optional) to taste
- 1/4 cup nutritional yeast flakes

Instructions:

1. Preheat oven to 375 degrees F.
2. In a large bowl, massage kale with olive oil until evenly coated. Season with salt and black pepper (optional) to taste.
3. Spread in an even layer on a baking sheet and bake for 10 minutes. Remove from oven and sprinkle with nutritional yeast flakes. Return to oven and bake for an additional 5-7 minutes, or until chips are crispy. Serve immediately!

Serving Size: 1/2 cup
Calories: 120

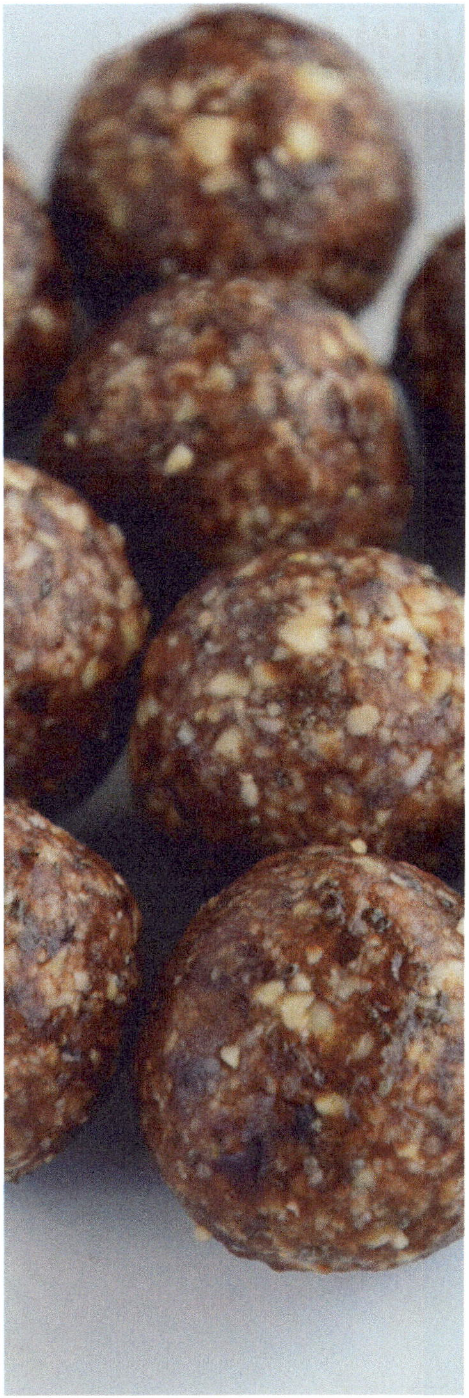

BLUEBERRY LEMON ENERGY BALLS

Ingredients:

- 1 cup old-fashioned oats
- 1/2 cup almond butter
- 1 teaspoon vanilla extract
- 1 cup fresh or frozen blueberries
- Zest of 1 lemon

Instructions:

1. In a large bowl, mix together oats, almond butter, and vanilla extract until well combined. Stir in blueberries and lemon zest.
2. Place mixture in the refrigerator for 30 minutes, or until firm.
3. Using wet hands, form mixture into small balls. Store in an airtight container in the refrigerator for up to 1 week.

Serving Size: 1 energy ball (Makes 12)
Calories: 110

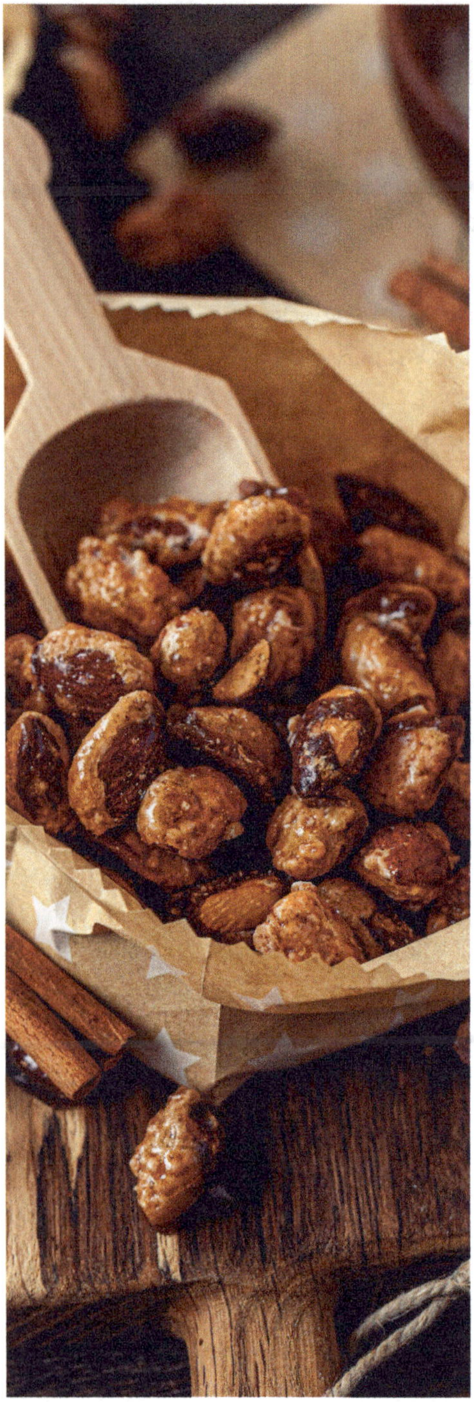

CINNAMON ROASTED ALMONDS

Ingredients:

- 1 cup raw almonds
- 1 tablespoon olive oil
- 1 teaspoon ground cinnamon

Instructions:

1. Preheat oven to 375 degrees F.
2. In a large bowl, toss together almonds and olive oil until evenly coated. Sprinkle with cinnamon and toss to combine.
3. Spread in an even layer on a baking sheet and roast for 10-12 minutes, or until almonds are fragrant and lightly browned. Serve immediately!

Serving Size: 1/4 cup
Calories: 140

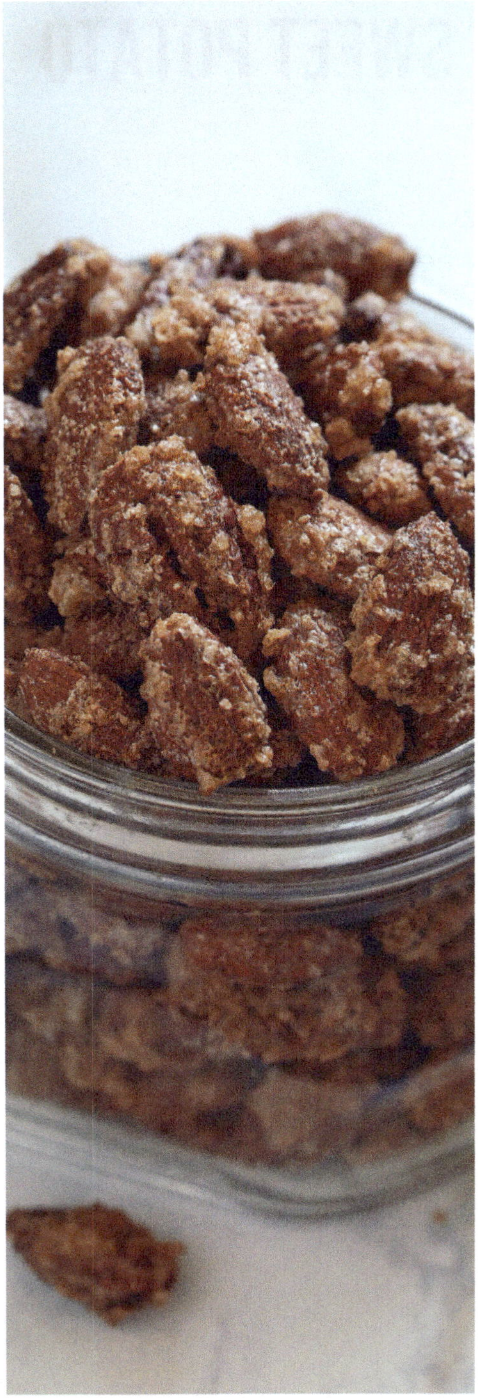

SPICED PECANS

Ingredients:

- 1 cup raw pecans
- 1 tablespoon olive oil
- 1 teaspoon chili powder
- 1/2 teaspoon ground cumin
- Salt (optional) and black pepper (optional) to taste

Instructions:

1. Preheat oven to 375 degrees F.
2. In a large bowl, toss together pecans, olive oil, chili powder, and cumin. Season with salt and black pepper (optional) to taste.
3. Spread in an even layer on a baking sheet and roast for 10-12 minutes, or until pecans are fragrant and lightly browned. Serve immediately!

Serving Size: 1/4 cup
Calories: 140

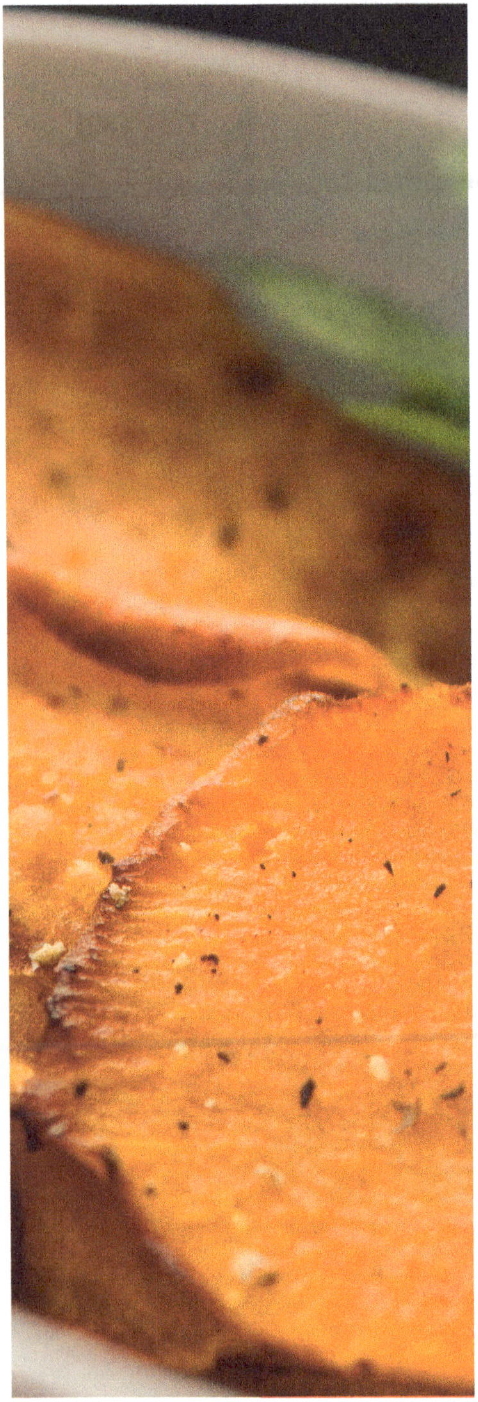

BAKED SWEET POTATO COINS

Ingredients:

- 3 large sweet potatoes, sliced into thin coins
- 1 tablespoon olive oil
- Salt (optional) and black pepper (optional) to taste

Instructions:

1. Preheat oven to 375 degrees F.
2. In a large bowl, toss together sweet potato coins and olive oil. Season with salt and black pepper (optional) to taste.
3. Spread in an even layer on a baking sheet and bake for 20-25 minutes, or until sweet potatoes are tender and lightly browned. Serve immediately!

Serving Size: 1/2 cup
Calories: 120

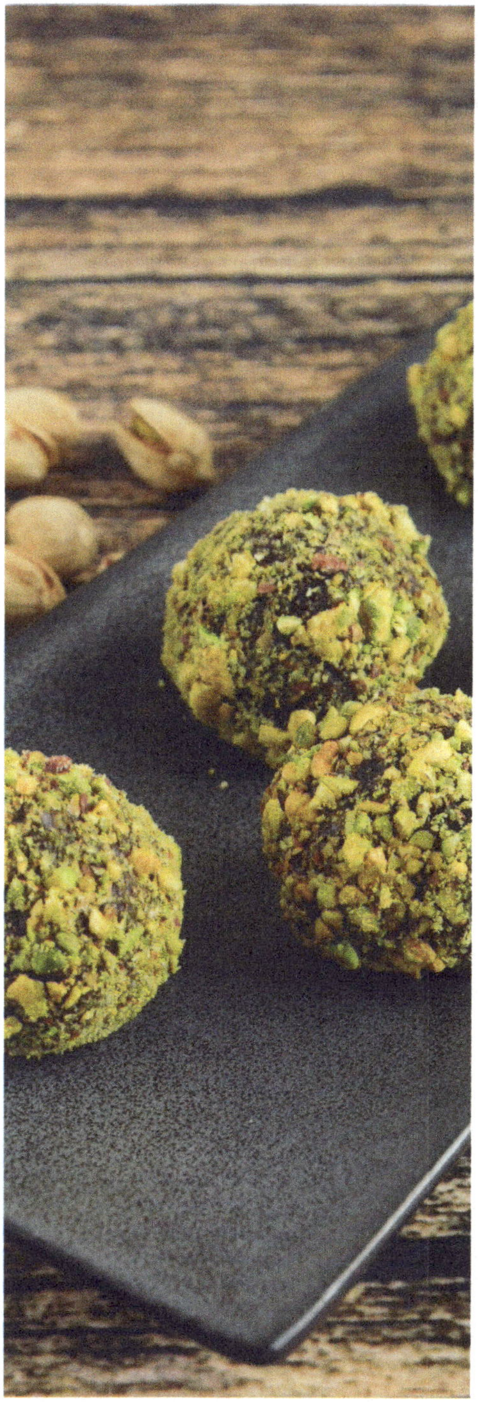

SAVORY DATE AND PISTACHIO BITES

Ingredients:

- 1 cup raw pistachios
- 1/2 cup pitted dates
- 1 teaspoon salt
- 1/4 teaspoon black pepper

Instructions:

1. In a food processor, combine pistachios, dates, salt, and black pepper. Process until mixture is finely chopped and sticky.
2. Using wet hands, form mixture into small balls. Store in an airtight container in the refrigerator for up to 1 week.

Serving Size: 1 bite (Makes 12)
Calories: 140

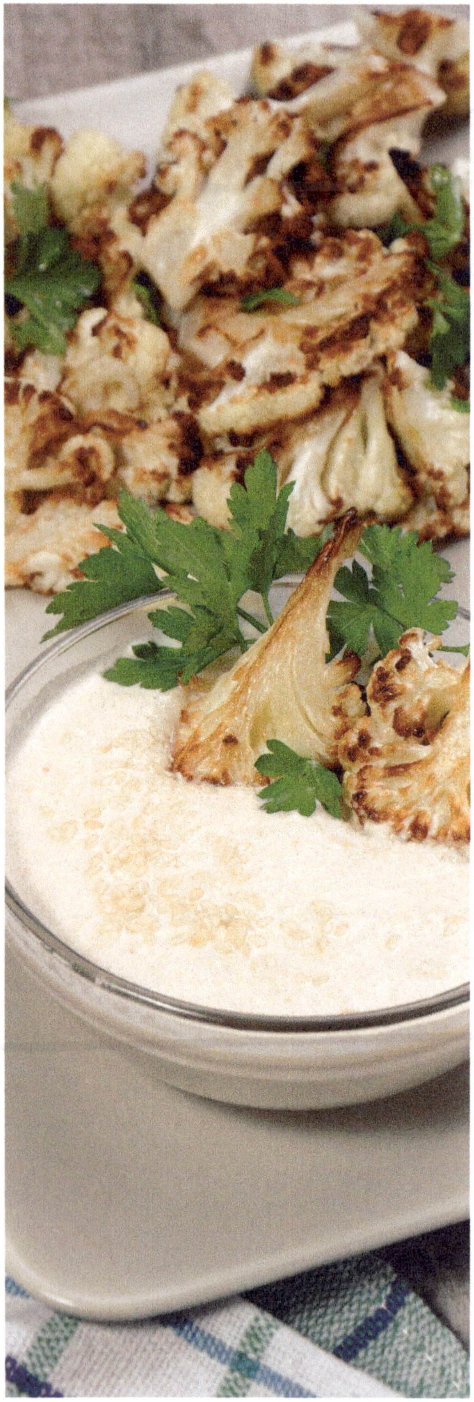

ROASTED CAULIFLOWER WITH TAHINI SAUCE

Ingredients:

- 1 head cauliflower, cut into florets
- 3 tablespoons olive oil
- Salt (optional) and black pepper (optional) to taste
- 1/4 cup tahini
- 1/4 cup water
- 2 tablespoons lemon juice
- 1 clove garlic, minced

Instructions:

1. Preheat oven to 375 degrees F.
2. In a large bowl, toss together cauliflower florets and olive oil. Season with salt and black pepper (optional) to taste.
3. Spread in an even layer on a baking sheet and roast for 25-30 minutes, or until cauliflower is tender and lightly browned.
4. In a small bowl, whisk together tahini, water, lemon juice, and garlic until smooth.
5. Serve roasted cauliflower warm, drizzled with tahini sauce.

Serving Size: 1/2 cup
Calories: 120

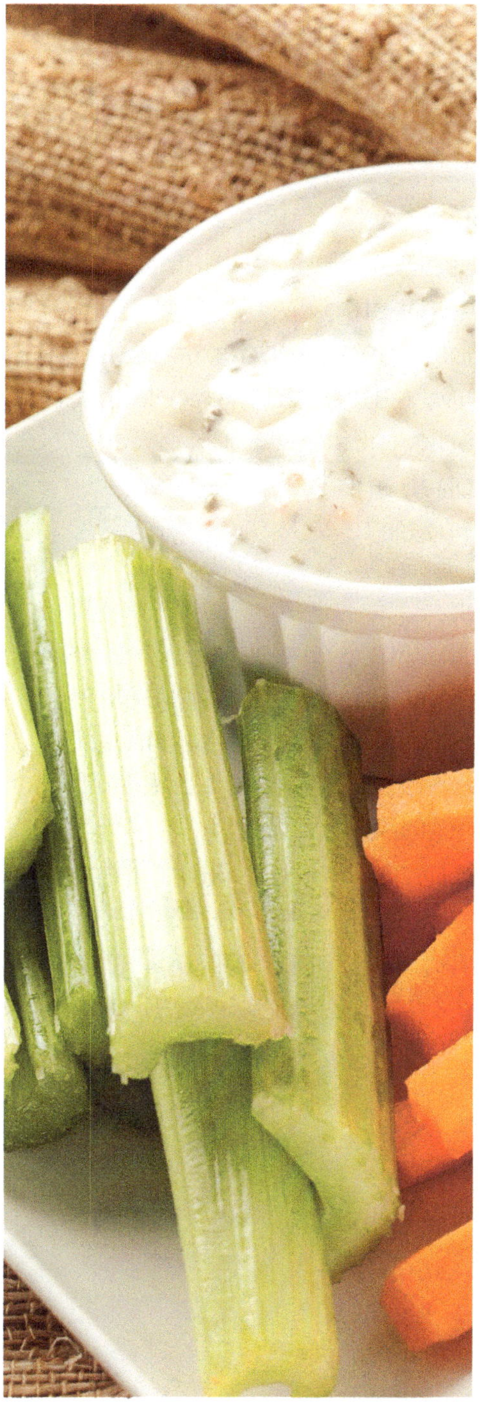

GARLIC WHITE BEAN DIP WITH CELERY STICKS

Ingredients:

- 1 (15-ounce) can white beans, drained and rinsed
- 2 cloves garlic, minced
- 1/4 cup tahini
- 1/4 cup water
- 2 tablespoons lemon juice
- Salt (optional) and black pepper (optional) to taste

Instructions:

1. In a food processor, combine white beans, garlic, tahini, water, and lemon juice. Season with salt and black pepper (optional) to taste. Process until mixture is smooth and creamy.
2. Serve dip with celery sticks or your favorite raw veggies!

Serving Size: 1/4 cup
Calories: 120

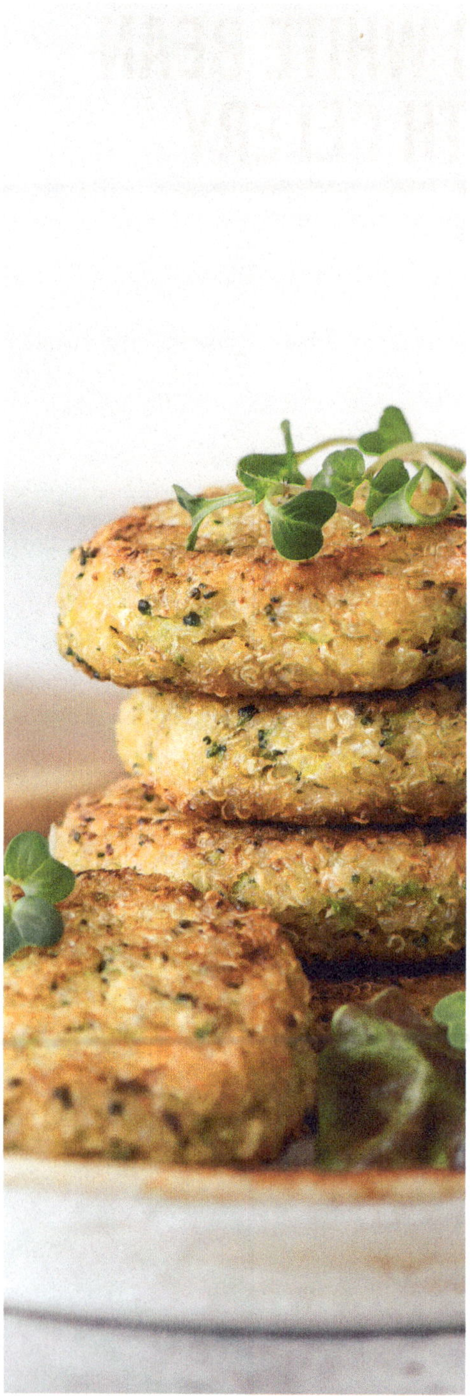

BAKED BROCCOLI-CHEDDAR QUINOA BITES

Ingredients:

- 1 cup cooked and cooled quinoa
- 1 large egg, beaten
- 1/4 cup shredded cheddar cheese
- 1/2 cup finely chopped broccoli florets
- 1 clove garlic, minced
- Salt (optional) and black pepper (optional) to taste

Instructions:

1. Preheat oven to 375 degrees F.
2. In a large bowl, mix together cooked quinoa, egg, cheddar cheese, broccoli, and garlic. Season with salt and black pepper (optional) to taste.
3. Using wet hands, form mixture into small balls. Place on a baking sheet lined with parchment paper and flatten slightly.
4. Bake for 12-15 minutes, or until quinoa bites are firm and golden brown. Serve immediately!

Serving Size: 2 quinoa bites
Calories: 120

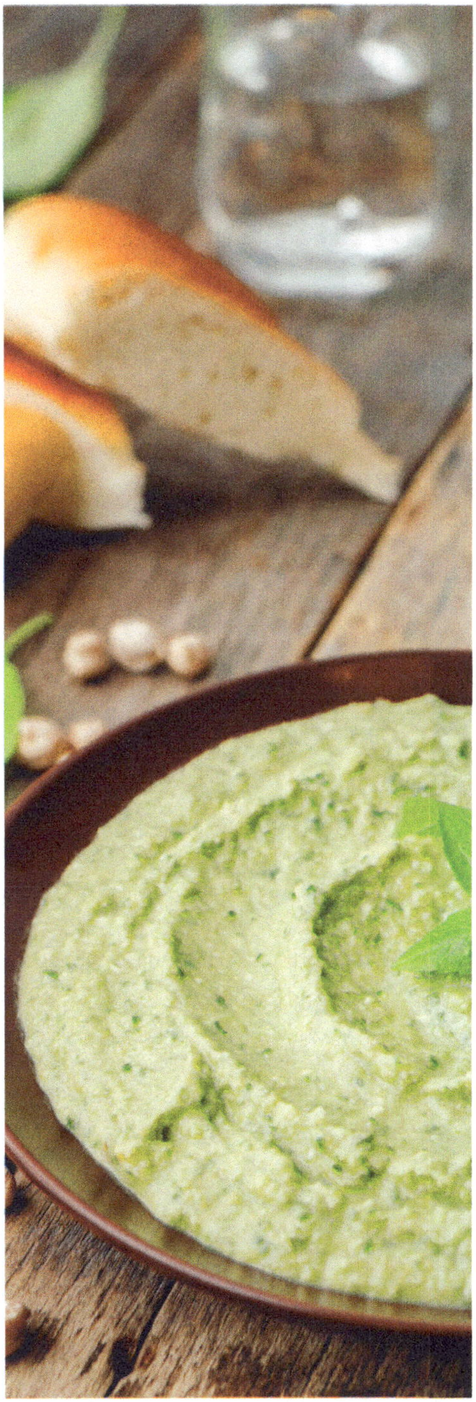

BASIL AND PESTO HUMMUS WITH PITA CHIPS

Ingredients:

- 1 (15-ounce) can chickpeas, drained and rinsed
- 1/4 cup tahini
- 2 cloves garlic, minced
- 3 tablespoons pesto
- 1/4 cup fresh basil leaves
- Salt (optional) and black pepper (optional) to taste

Instructions:

1. In a food processor, combine chickpeas, tahini, garlic, pesto, and basil leaves. Season with salt and black pepper (optional) to taste. Process until mixture is smooth and creamy.
2. Serve hummus with pita chips or your favorite raw veggies!

Serving Size: 1/4 cup
Calories: 100

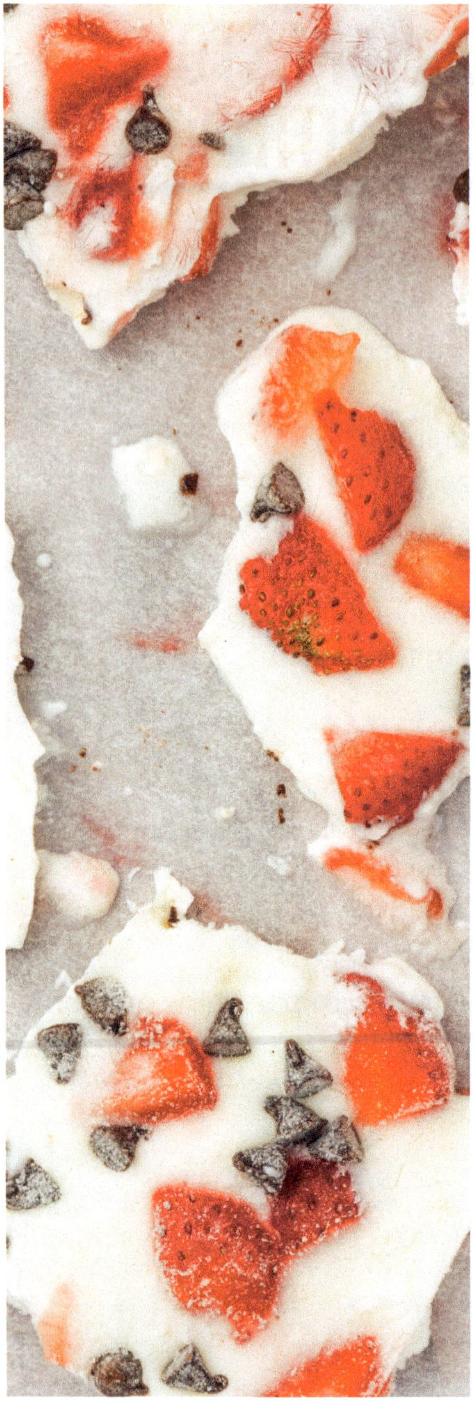

STRAWBERRY-CHOCOLATE GREEK YOGURT BARK

Ingredients:

- 2 cups plain Greek yogurt
- 1 cup strawberries, finely chopped
- 1/4 cup dark chocolate chips

Instructions:

1. Line a baking sheet with parchment paper.
2. In a medium bowl, mix together Greek yogurt, strawberries, and chocolate chips until completely combined.
3. Spread mixture in an even layer on the prepared baking sheet. Freeze for 2 hours, or until frozen solid.
4. Break into pieces and enjoy! Store leftovers in the freezer in an airtight container for up to 2 months.

Serving Size: 1 piece (Makes 12)
Calories: 110

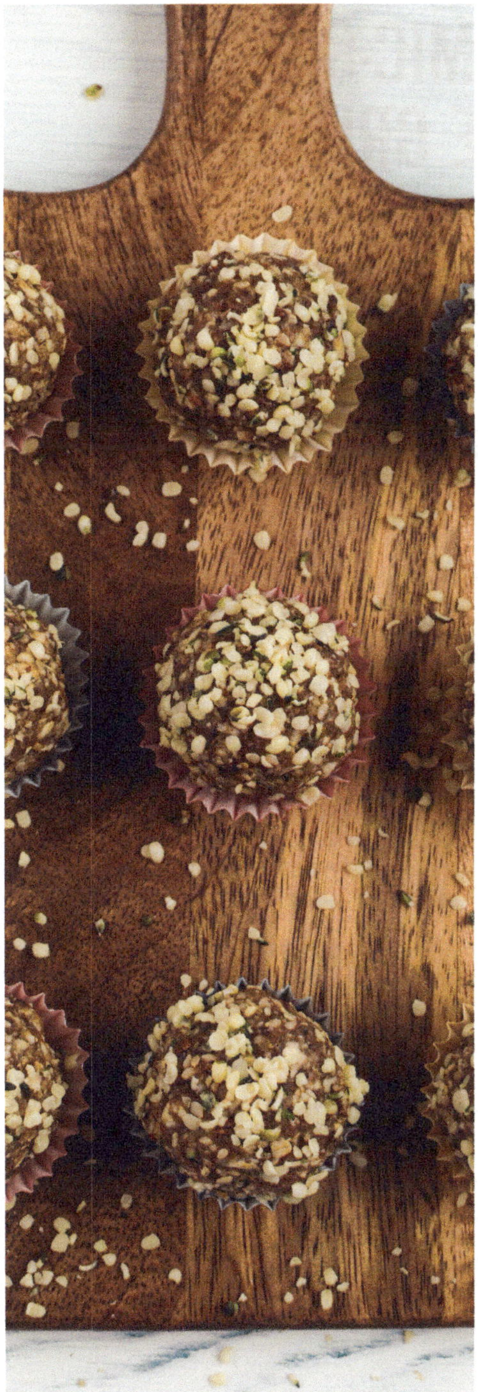

APRICOT-GINGER ENERGY BALLS

Ingredients:

- 1 cup dried apricots, finely chopped
- 1/2 cup almonds, finely chopped
- 1/4 cup ground flaxseed
- 1 teaspoon grated ginger

Instructions:

1. In a large bowl, mix together all ingredients until completely combined.
2. Using wet hands, form mixture into small balls. Store in an airtight container in the fridge for up to 1 week.

Serving Size: 1 ball (Makes 12)
Calories: 120

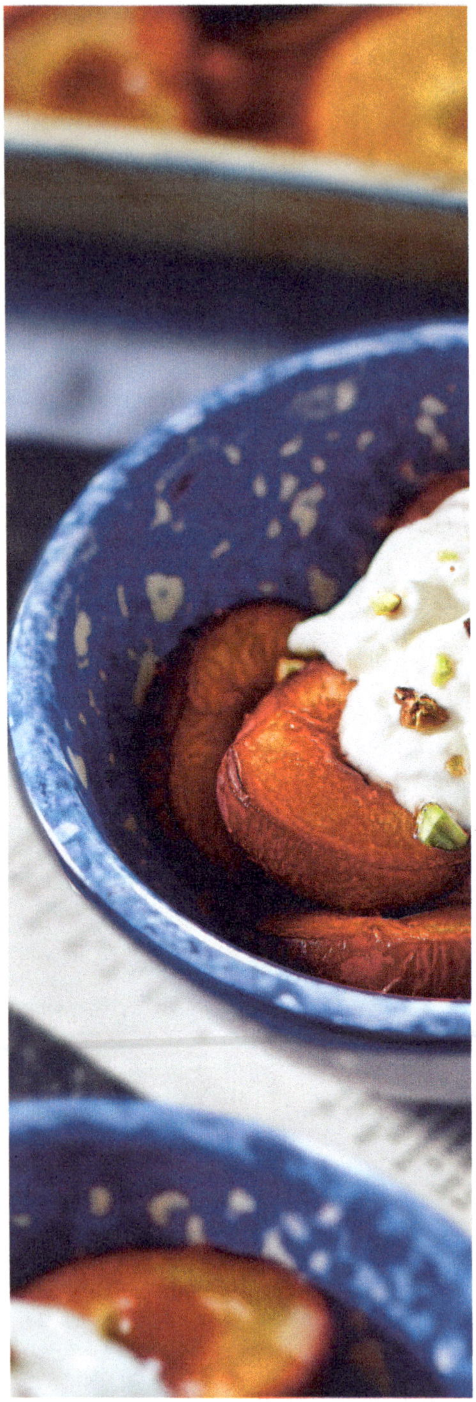

BALSAMIC-GOAT CHEESE GRILLED PLUMS

Ingredients:

- 4 ripe plums, halved and pitted
- 2 tablespoons balsamic vinegar
- 1 tablespoon olive oil
- Salt (optional) and black pepper (optional) to taste
- 2 ounces goat cheese, crumbled

Instructions:

1. Preheat grill to medium-high heat.
2. In a small bowl, whisk together balsamic vinegar, olive oil, salt, and black pepper (optional).
3. Grill plum halves for 2-3 minutes per side, or until slightly charred. Remove from grill and drizzle with balsamic vinegar mixture. Top with crumbled goat cheese and serve immediately!

Serving Size: 1/2 plum
Calories: 130

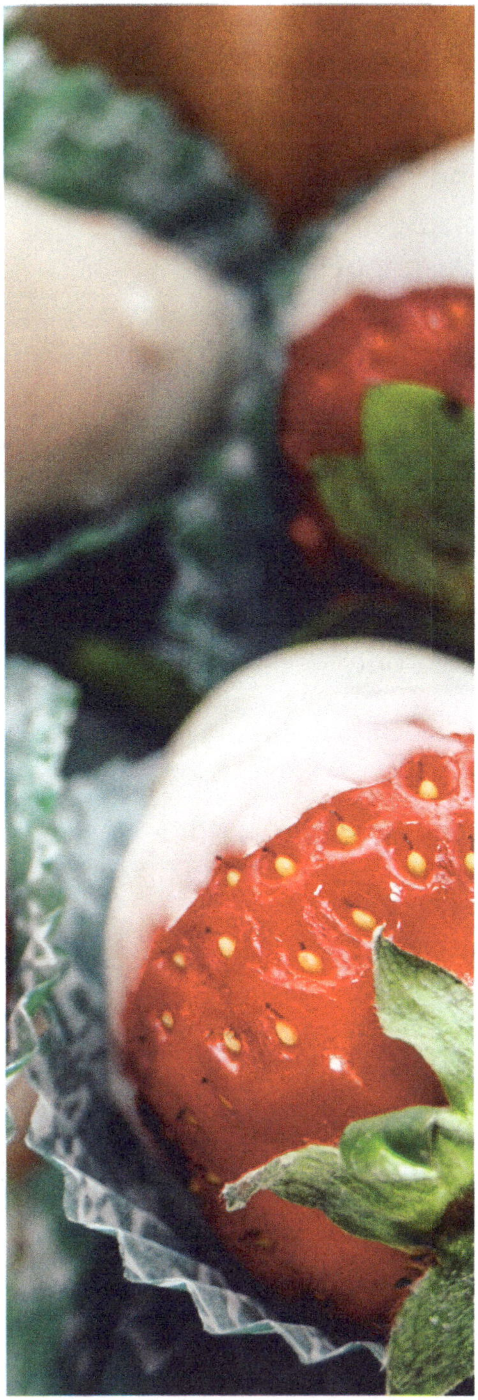

FROZEN YOGURT-COVERED STRAWBERRIES

Ingredients:

- 1 pound fresh strawberries, hulled and halved
- 1 cup plain Greek yogurt

Instructions:

1. Line a baking sheet with parchment paper.
2. In a medium bowl, mix together Greek yogurt and strawberries until well combined.
3. Using a small spoon or your fingers, coat each strawberry half with yogurt. Place on the prepared baking sheet and freeze for 2 hours, or until frozen solid.
4. Enjoy as is or store in the freezer in an airtight container for up to 2 months.

Serving Size: 1 strawberry (Makes 24)
Calories: 40

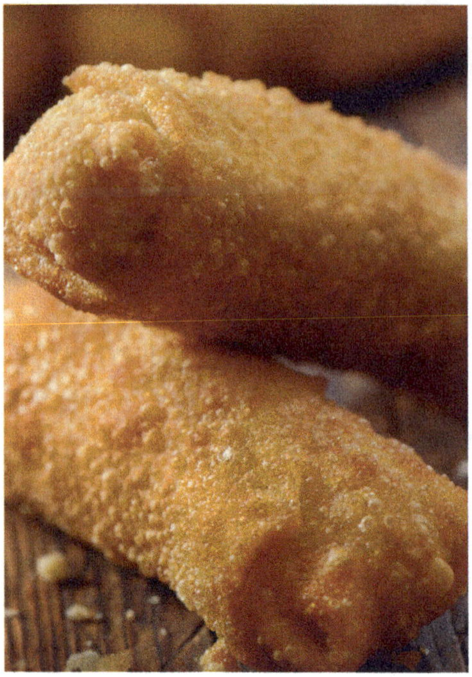

SOUTHWEST EGG ROLLS

Ingredients:

- 1 tablespoon olive oil
- 1/2 cup onion, diced
- 1/4 cup bell pepper, diced
- 1/2 teaspoon ground cumin
- Salt (optional) and black pepper (optional) to taste
- 1 (15-ounce) can black beans, drained and rinsed
- 1/2 cup frozen corn kernels, thawed
- 1/4 cup prepared salsa
- 1/2 cup shredded cheddar cheese
- 6 egg roll wrappers

Instructions:

1. Preheat oven to 375 degrees F.
2. In a large skillet, heat olive oil over medium heat. Add onion and bell pepper and cook until softened, about 5 minutes. Stir in cumin, salt, and black pepper (optional) and cook for 1 minute.
3. Add black beans, corn, salsa, and cheddar cheese to the skillet. Mix until well combined and heated through.
4. Place egg roll wrappers on a work surface. Spoon about 1/4 cup of the bean mixture into the center of each wrapper. Wet the edges of the wrapper with water and roll up, sealing tightly.
5. Place egg rolls on a baking sheet lined with parchment paper. Bake for 15-20 minutes, or until golden brown and crispy! Serve with your favorite dipping sauce.

Serving Size: 1 egg roll
Calories: 210

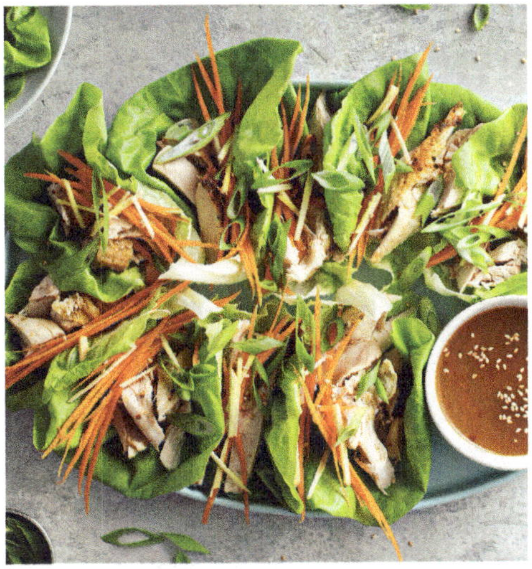

ASIAN WRAPS

Ingredients:

- 1/4 cup tahini
- 1/4 cup soy sauce
- 1 tablespoon sugar-free honey substitute
- 1 teaspoon rice vinegar
- 1 clove garlic, minced
- 6 ounces extra-firm tofu, drained and pressed

Instructions:

1. In a small bowl, whisk together tahini, soy sauce, honey substitute, rice vinegar, and garlic until well combined. Set aside.
2. Cut tofu into small cubes and place in a medium bowl. Pour half of the tahini mixture over the tofu and mix until well coated.
3. Preheat grill to medium-high heat.
4. Spray a grilling basket with cooking spray (optional). Add tofu to the basket and grill for 15-20 minutes, or until tofu is slightly charred and crisp. Remove from grill and let cool for 5 minutes.
5. To assemble wraps, place 3-4 grilled tofu cubes on a lettuce leaf. Top with shredded carrots, red pepper strips, and green onions. Drizzle with remaining tahini mixture and roll up. Serve immediately!

Serving Size: 1 wrap (Makes 4)
Calories: 350

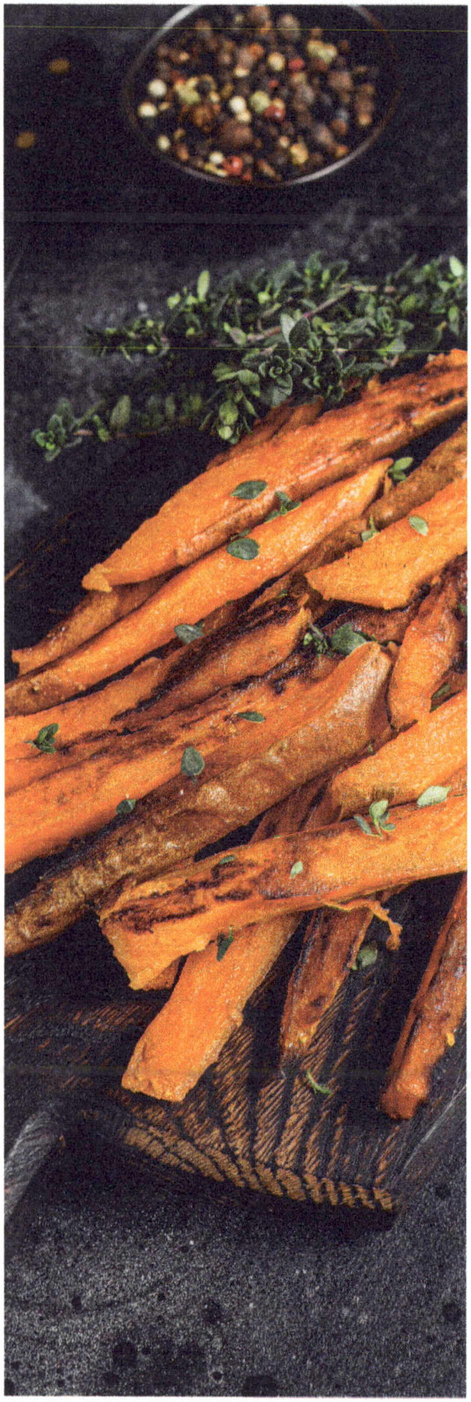

ROASTED SWEET POTATO WEDGES

Ingredients:

- 2 large sweet potatoes, cut into wedges
- 1 tablespoon olive oil
- Salt (optional) and black pepper (optional) to taste

Instructions:

1. Preheat oven to 400 degrees F.
2. In a large bowl, toss together sweet potatoes and olive oil until well coated. Season with salt (optional) and black pepper (optional) to taste.
3. Spread sweet potatoes in an even layer on a baking sheet lined with parchment paper. Roast for 25-30 minutes, or until tender and slightly browned. Serve immediately!

Serving Size: 1/2 cup
Calories: 110

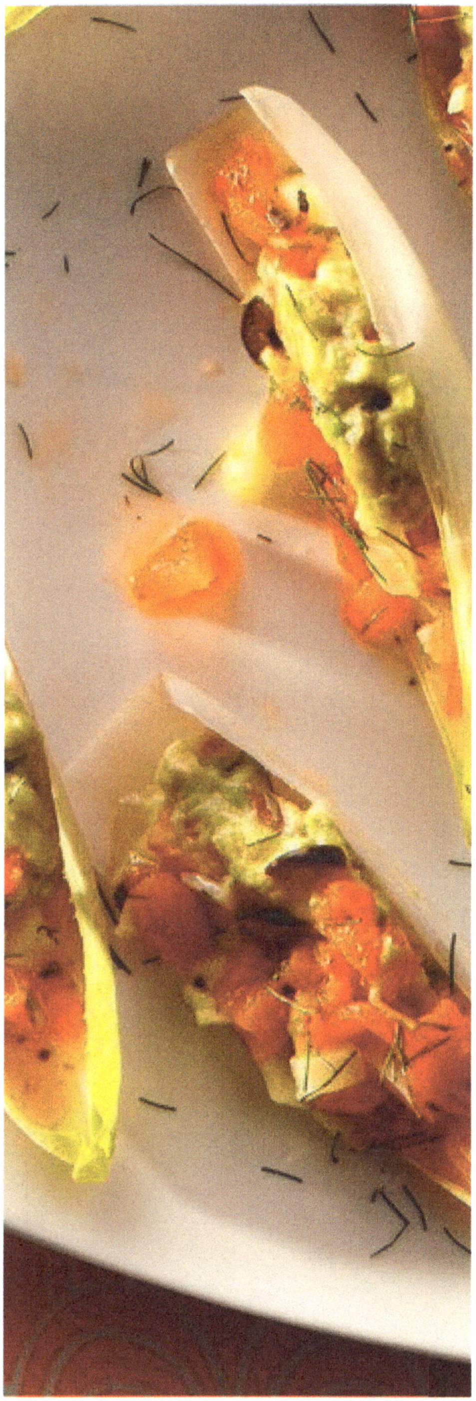

AVOCADO ENDIVE CUPS WITH SALSA

Ingredients:

- 1 large avocado, diced
- 1/4 cup prepared salsa
- 2 heads Belgian endive, leaves separated

Instructions:

1. In a small bowl, mix together avocado and salsa until well combined.
2. Spoon avocado mixture into the center of each endive leaf. Serve immediately!

Serving Size: 2 cups (Makes 12)
Calories: 60

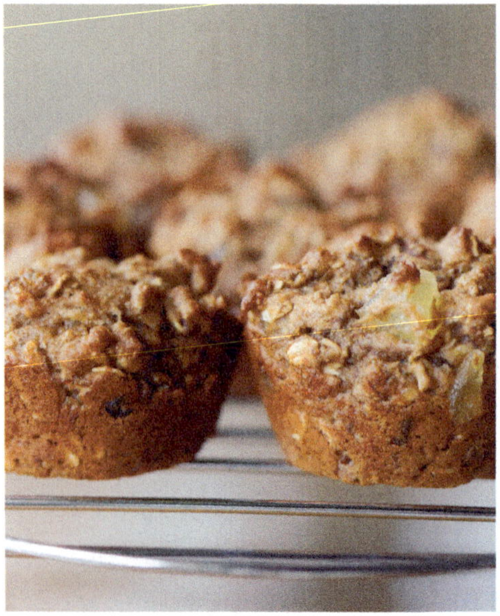

MINI MORNING GLORY MUFFINS

Ingredients:

- 1 cup whole wheat flour
- 1 teaspoon baking powder
- 1/4 teaspoon baking soda
- 1/4 teaspoon salt (optional)
- 1 teaspoon ground cinnamon
- 1/2 cup unsweetened applesauce
- 1/4 cup sugar-free honey substitute
- 1 egg, beaten

Instructions:

1. Preheat oven to 350 degrees F. Line a mini muffin tin with paper liners and set aside.
2. In a large bowl, whisk together whole wheat flour, baking powder, baking soda, salt (optional), and cinnamon.
3. In a separate bowl, mix together applesauce, honey substitute, and egg. Pour wet ingredients into dry ingredients and mix until well combined.
4. Fill each muffin cup about 3/4 full with batter. Bake for 12-15 minutes, or until a toothpick inserted into the center comes out clean. Let cool for 5 minutes before removing from tin. Serve immediately!

Serving Size: 1 muffin (Makes 24)
Calories: 60

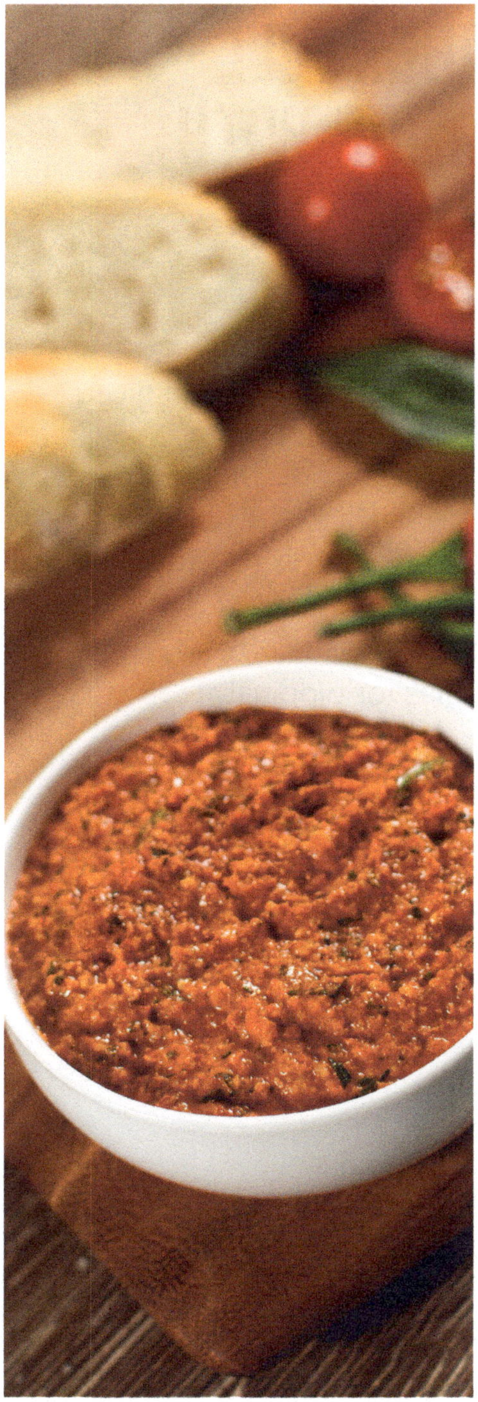

ROASTED RED PEPPER TAPENADE

Ingredients:

- 1/2 cup pitted kalamata olives
- 1/2 cup roasted red peppers
- 1 clove garlic, minced
- 1 tablespoon olive oil
- Salt (optional) and black pepper (optional) to taste

Instructions:

1. In a food processor or blender, combine all ingredients and blend until smooth. Season with salt (optional) and black pepper (optional) to taste.
2. Serve with crackers, whole wheat bread, or vegetables for dipping!

Serving Size: 2 tablespoons (Makes 1/2 cup)
Calories: 60

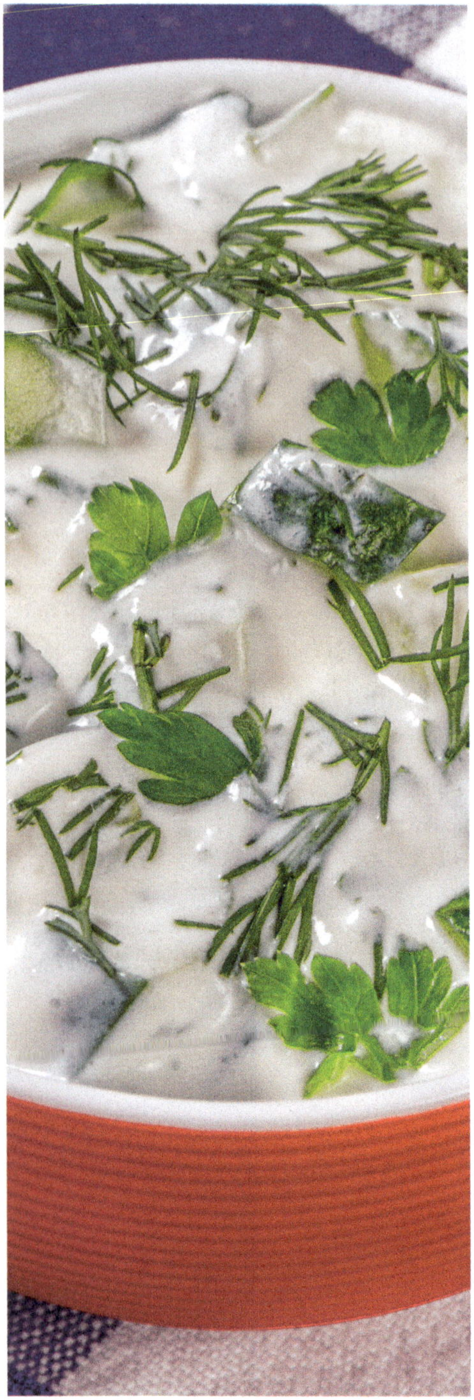

CUCUMBER DILL YOGURT DIP WITH VEGETABLES

Ingredients:

- 1 cup plain yogurt
- 1 large cucumber, peeled and diced
- 1/4 cup fresh dill, chopped

Instructions:

1. In a medium bowl, mix together yogurt, cucumber, and dill until well combined.
2. Serve with crackers, whole wheat bread, or vegetables for dipping!

Serving Size: 2 tablespoons (Makes 1 cup)
Calories: 25

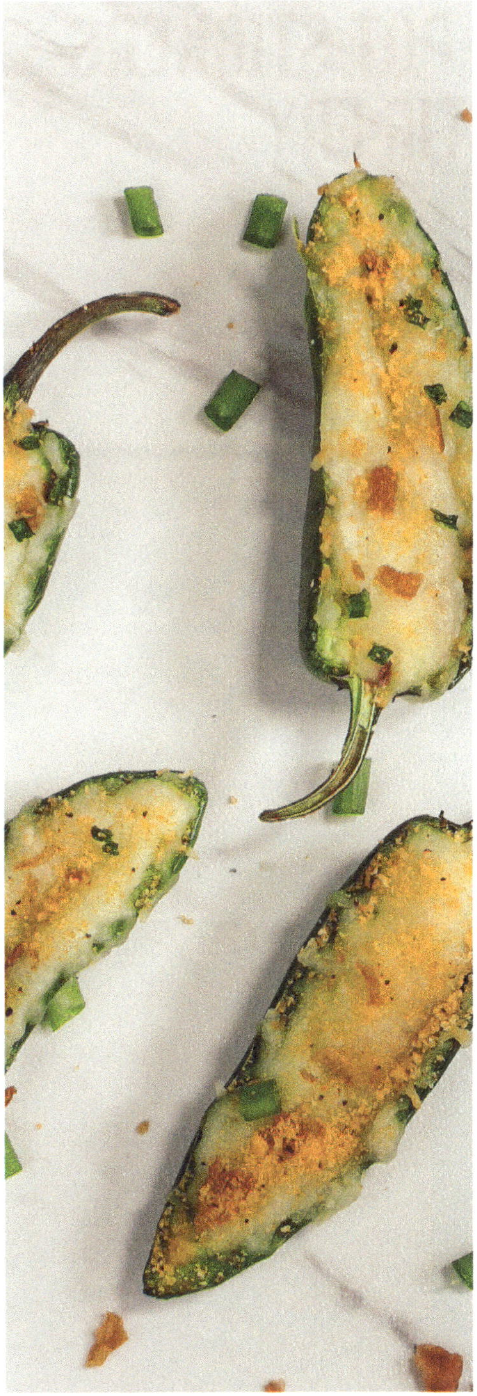

JALAPENO POPPERS

Ingredients:

- 6 large jalapeno peppers, halved lengthwise and seeds removed
- 1/4 cup fat-free cream cheese
- 3 tablespoons shredded low-fat cheddar cheese

Instructions:

1. Preheat oven to 350 degrees F.
2. In a small bowl, mix together cream cheese and cheddar cheese until well combined.
3. Spoon mixture into the center of each jalapeno half. Place on a baking sheet lined with parchment paper and bake for 15-20 minutes, or until peppers are tender and cheese is melted and bubbly. Serve immediately!

Serving Size: 1 popper (Makes 12)
Calories: 25

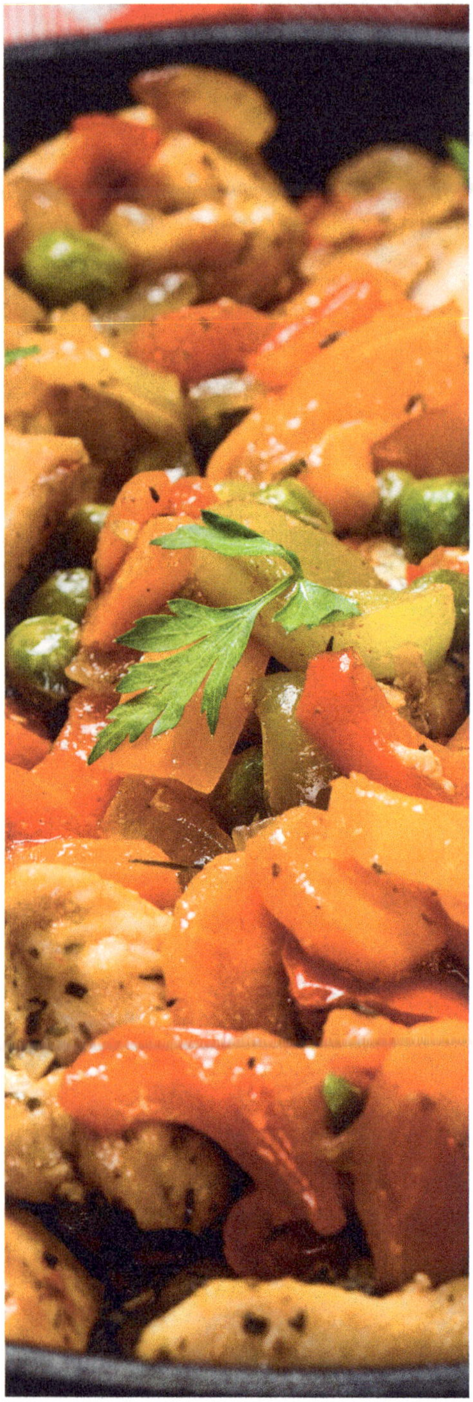

BAKED POT STICKERS WITH STIR-FRY SAUCE

Ingredients:

For the pot stickers:

- 1/2 pound ground chicken
- 1/4 cup shredded carrots
- 1/4 cup chopped green onions
- 3 cloves garlic, minced
- 1 teaspoon freshly grated ginger
- 1 tablespoon soy sauce
- 1 teaspoon sesame oil
- 24 wonton wrappers
- Cooking spray

For the stir-fry sauce:

- 1/4 cup chicken broth
- 1 tablespoon low-sodium soy sauce
- 1 tablespoon rice vinegar
- 1 teaspoon sesame oil
- 1 clove garlic, minced

Instructions:

1. Preheat oven to 375 degrees F.
2. In a large bowl, mix together ground chicken, carrots, green onions, garlic, ginger, soy sauce, and sesame oil until well combined.
3. To assemble the pot stickers, spoon 1 tablespoon of filling into the center of each wonton wrapper. Wet the edges of the wrapper with water and fold over to form a triangle, pressing to seal. Place on a baking sheet lined with parchment paper and lightly spray with cooking spray. Bake for 12-15 minutes, or until golden brown and crispy.
4. While pot stickers are baking, prepare stir-fry sauce by whisking together chicken broth, soy sauce, rice vinegar, sesame oil, and garlic in a small bowl.
5. Serve pot stickers with stir-fry sauce for dipping!

Serving Size: 2 pot stickers (Makes 24)
Calories: 100

CHAPTER THREE:
Breakfasts

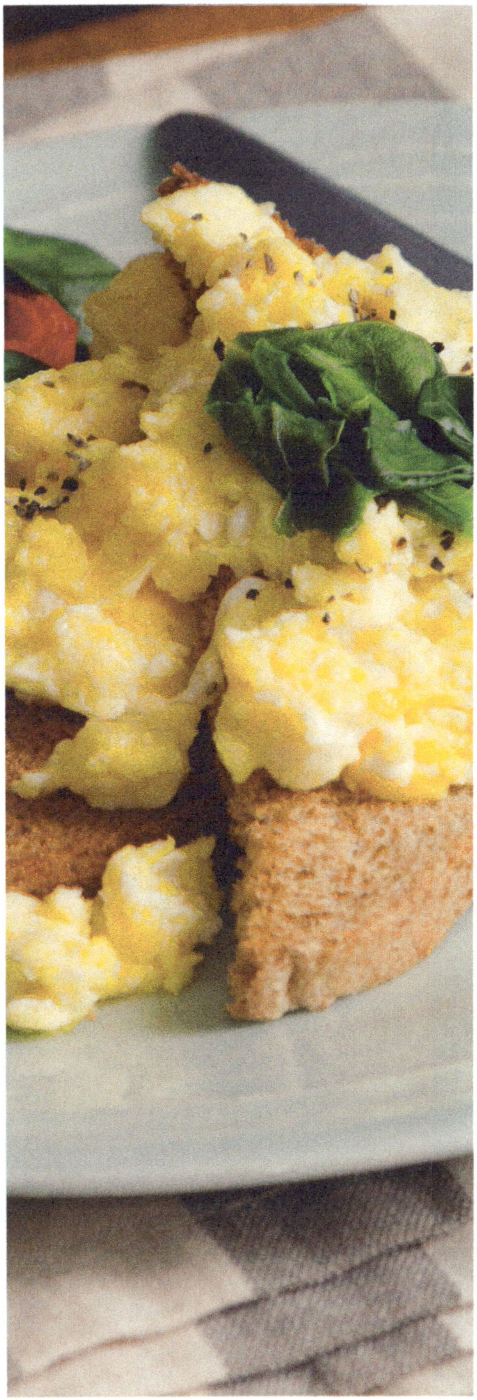

SPINACH AND EGG SCRAMBLE WITH RASPBERRIES ON TOAST

Ingredients:

- 1 tablespoon olive oil
- 2 cups spinach, chopped
- 4 eggs, beaten
- Salt (optional) and black pepper (optional) to taste
- 1/2 cup raspberries, fresh or frozen
- 2 slices whole wheat bread, toasted

Instructions:

1. In a large skillet over medium heat, heat olive oil. Add spinach and cook until wilted.
2. Add eggs and scramble until cooked through. Season with salt and black pepper (optional) to taste.
3. Stir in raspberries and remove from heat. Divide scramble evenly between toast slices and serve immediately!

Serving Size: 1 breakfast sandwich
Calories: 390

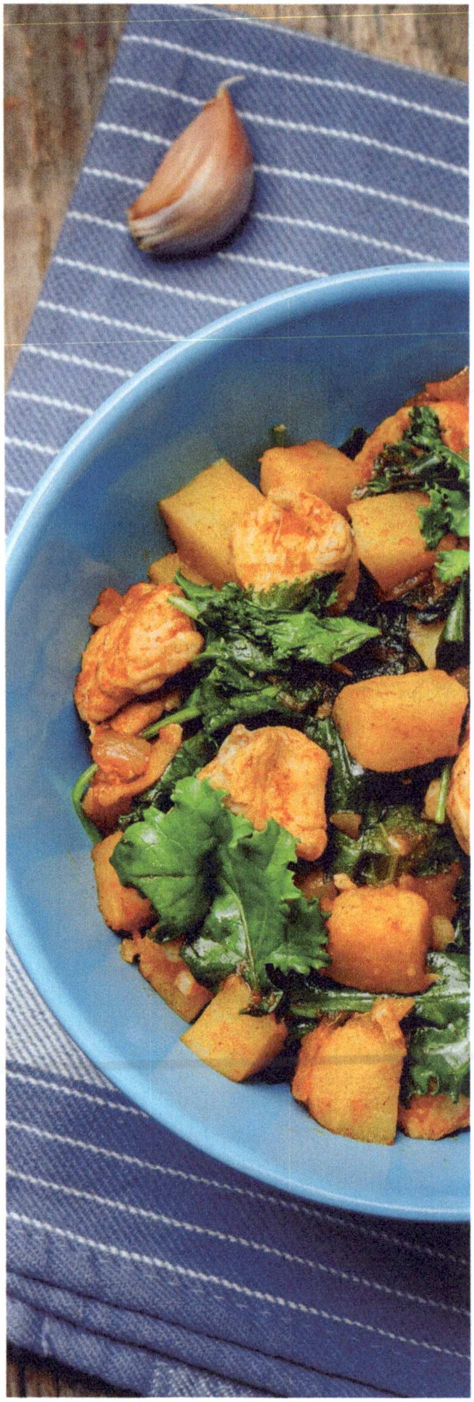

SWEET POTATO AND CHICKEN SAUSAGE HASH

Ingredients:

- 1 tablespoon olive oil
- 2 cups diced sweet potato
- 1/4 cup diced onion
- 3 cloves garlic, minced
- 8 ounces chicken sausage, sliced into bite-sized pieces
- Salt (optional) and black pepper (optional) to taste

Instructions:

1. In a large skillet over medium heat, heat olive oil. Add sweet potato, onion, and garlic and cook until all vegetables are soft.
2. Add chicken sausage and continue to cook until browned. Season with salt and black pepper (optional) to taste. Serve immediately!

Serving Size: 1 bowl of hash
Calories: 410

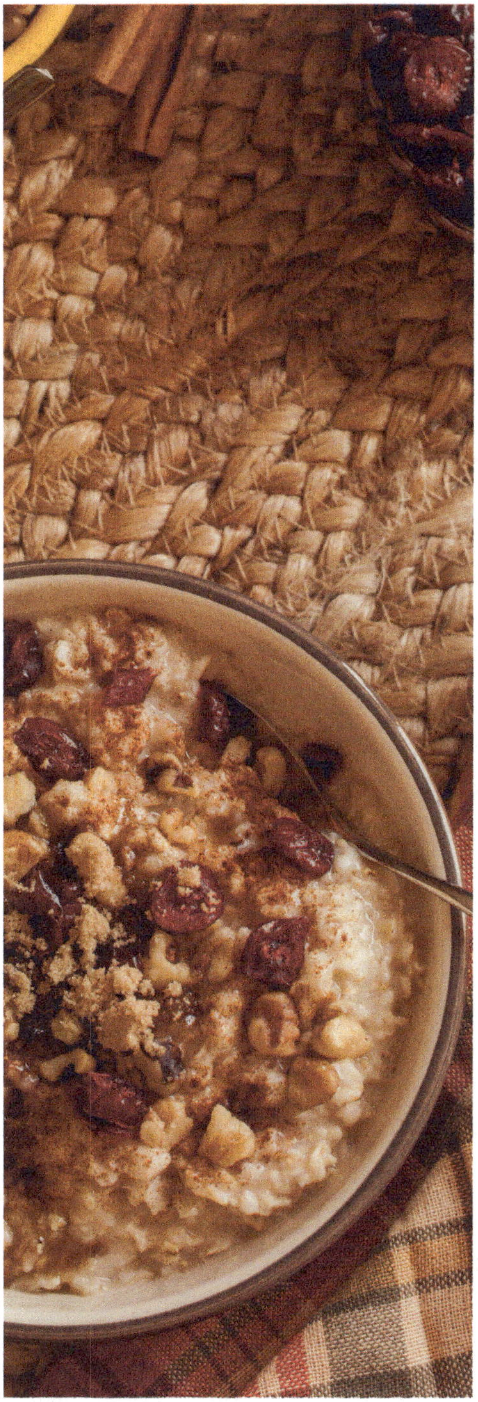

PUMPKIN SPICE OATMEAL WITH DRIED CRANBERRIES

Ingredients:

- 1 cup milk (1% dairy, almond, or soy)
- 1 cup water
- 1 cup quick-cooking oats
- 2 tablespoons canned pumpkin puree
- 1 teaspoon pumpkin pie spice
- 1/4 cup dried cranberries

Instructions:

1. In a medium saucepan over medium heat, bring milk and water to a boil.
2. Stir in oats, pumpkin puree, and pumpkin pie spice. Cook for 1 minute, or until oats are cooked through.
3. Remove from heat and stir in dried cranberries. Serve immediately!

Serving Size: 1 bowl of oatmeal
Calories: 320

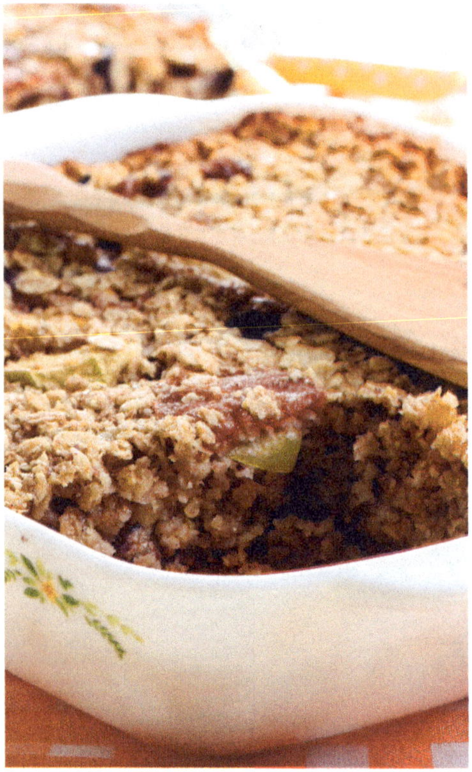

BAKED OATMEAL WITH PEARS AND PECANS

Ingredients:

- 2 cups old-fashioned oats
- 1/4 cup Stevia
- 1 teaspoon baking powder
- 1 teaspoon cinnamon
- 1/4 teaspoon salt (optional)
- 2 cups milk (1% dairy, almond, or soy)
- 1 egg, beaten
- 1 tablespoon vanilla extract
- 2 pears, peeled and diced
- 1/4 cup chopped pecans

Instructions:

1. Preheat oven to 375 degrees F.
2. In a large bowl, mix together oats, Stevia, baking powder, cinnamon, and salt (optional).
3. Stir in milk, egg, and vanilla extract until well combined. Fold in pears and pecans.
4. Pour into a greased 9×13 inch baking dish and bake for 25-30 minutes, or until oatmeal is set and golden brown. Serve immediately!

Serving Size: 1 square of oatmeal
Calories: 320

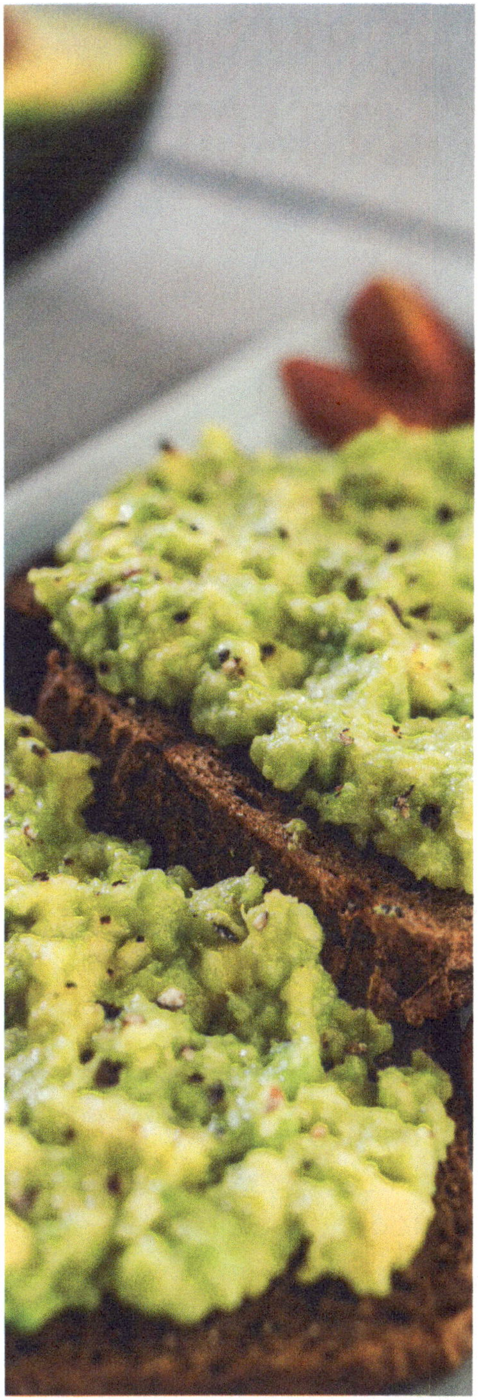

MEYER LEMON AVOCADO TOAST

Ingredients:

- 1 avocado, diced
- 1 Meyer lemon, juiced
- Salt (optional) and black pepper (optional) to taste
- 2 slices whole wheat bread, toasted

Instructions:

1. In a small bowl, mix together avocado and Meyer lemon juice. Season with salt and black pepper (optional) to taste.
2. Spread avocado mixture on toast and serve immediately!

Serving Size: 1 avocado toast
Calories: 290

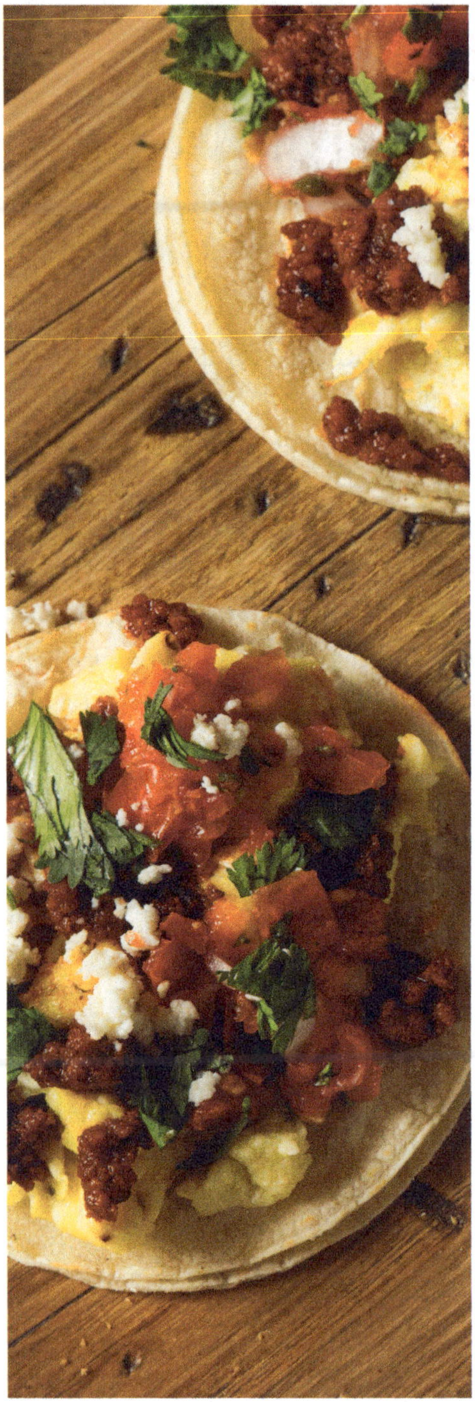

BEAN AND BACON BREAKFAST TACOS

Ingredients:

- 4 bacon strips, diced
- 1/2 cup diced onion
- 3 cloves garlic, minced
- 1 (15-ounce) can black beans, rinsed and drained
- 8 eggs, beaten
- Salt (optional) and black pepper (optional) to taste
- 8 (6-inch) whole wheat tortillas.

Instructions:

1. In a large skillet over medium heat, cook bacon until crisp. Remove with a slotted spoon and set aside on a paper towel-lined plate.
2. Add onion and garlic to the bacon fat and cook until softened. Stir in black beans and cook for 2 minutes.
3. Add eggs and scramble until cooked through. Season with salt and black pepper (optional) to taste.
4. Divide egg mixture evenly between tortillas and top with bacon. Serve immediately!

Serving Size: 2 tacos
Calories: 440

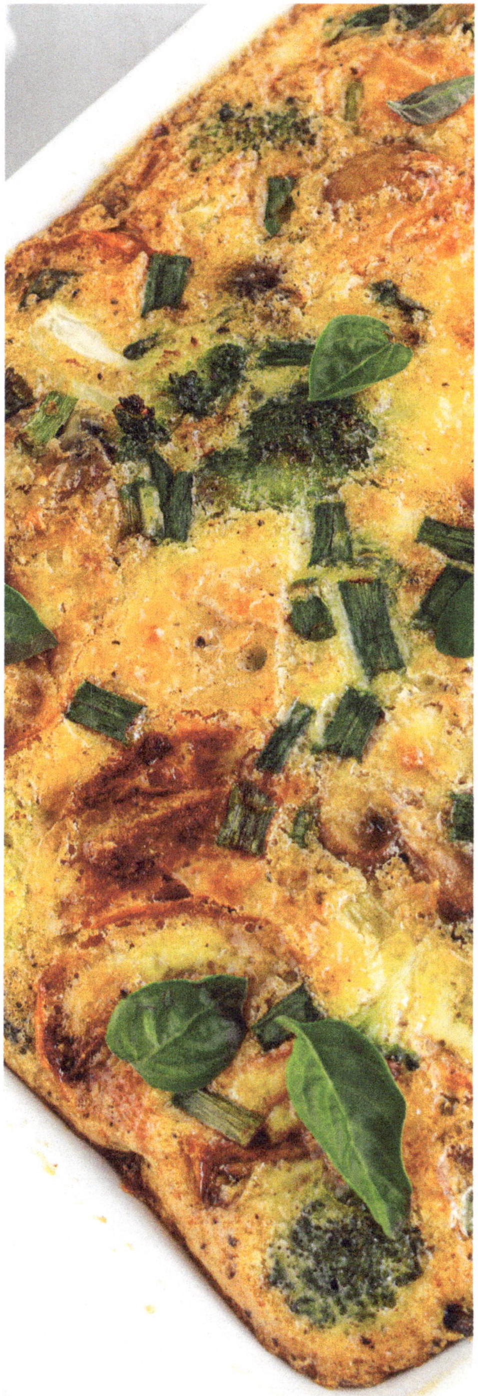

SAUSAGE, EGG, AND CHEESE BREAKFAST CASSEROLE

Ingredients:

- 1 pound sausage, cooked and crumbled
- 8 eggs, beaten
- 1/2 cup milk (1% dairy, almond, or soy)
- 1 tablespoon mustard
- 1/4 teaspoon salt (optional)
- Black pepper (optional) to taste
- 2 cups shredded cheddar cheese

Instructions:

1. Preheat oven to 350 degrees F.
2. In a large bowl, mix together sausage, eggs, milk, mustard, salt (optional), and black pepper (optional).
3. Pour into a greased 9×13 inch baking dish and sprinkle with cheddar cheese. Bake for 25-30 minutes, or until casserole is set and golden brown. Serve immediately!

Serving Size: 1 piece of casserole
Calories: 490

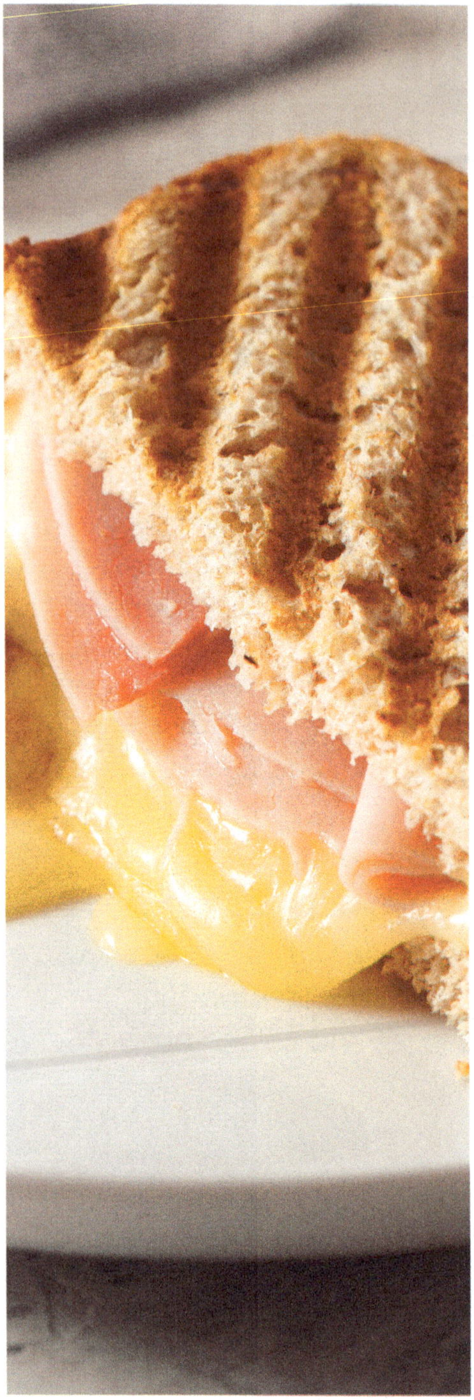

HAM AND CHEESE BREAKFAST SLIDERS

Ingredients:

- 1 (12-ounce) package whole wheat rolls, sliced in half horizontally
- 1/4 cup yellow onion, diced
- 1/4 cup red pepper, diced
- 1/4 cup green pepper, diced
- 8 ounces ham, diced
- 8 ounces Swiss cheese, shredded
- 1/2 cup (1 stick) butter, melted
- 1 tablespoon poppy seeds

Instructions:

1. Preheat oven to 375 degrees F.
2. In a large bowl, mix together onion, red pepper, green pepper, ham, Swiss cheese, and butter.
3. Arrange the bottom half of the rolls in a single layer on a greased 9×13 inch baking dish. Top with the ham and cheese mixture and then the top half of the rolls. Brush with additional butter and sprinkle with poppy seeds.
4. Bake for 10-15 minutes, or until bread is toasted and cheese is melted. Serve immediately!

Serving Size: 1 slider
Calories: 340

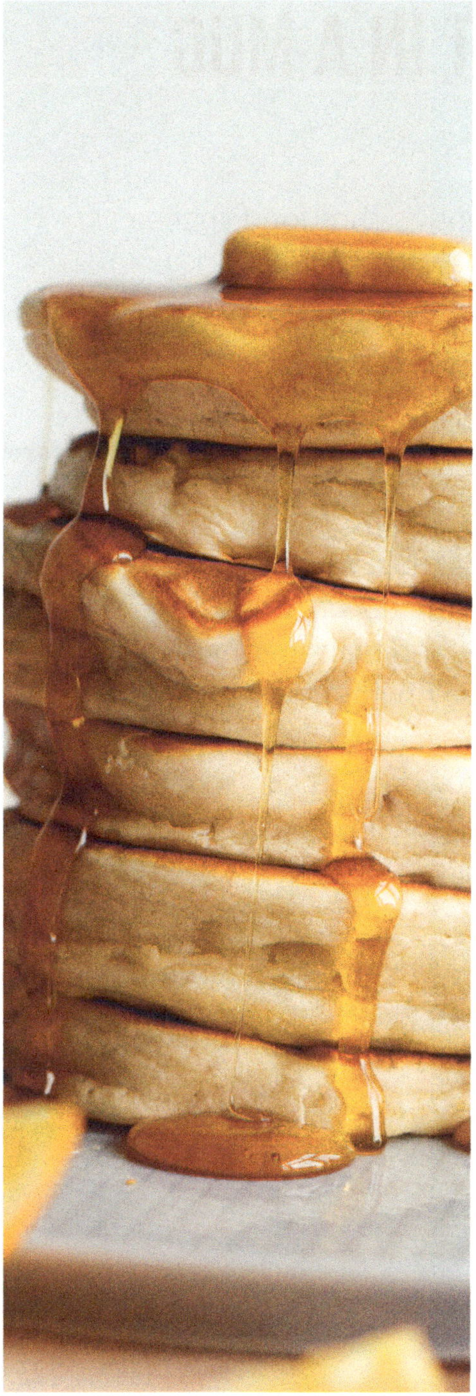

GREEK YOGURT PANCAKES

Ingredients:

- 1 cup whole wheat flour
- 2 teaspoons baking powder
- 1/4 teaspoon baking soda
- 1/4 teaspoon salt (optional)
- 1 tablespoon Stevia
- 1 egg, beaten
- 1 cup Greek yogurt (plain or vanilla)
- 1/2 cup milk (1% dairy, almond, or soy)

Instructions:

1. In a large bowl, mix together flour, baking powder, baking soda, salt (optional), and Stevia.
2. In a separate bowl, whisk together egg, yogurt, and milk. Stir into the dry ingredients until just combined.
3. Grease a griddle or skillet over medium heat and drop batter by the 1/4 cup onto the surface. Cook for 2-3 minutes per side, or until golden brown and cooked through. Serve immediately with your favorite toppings (syrup, fruit, etc.)!

Serving Size: 2 pancakes
Calories: 340

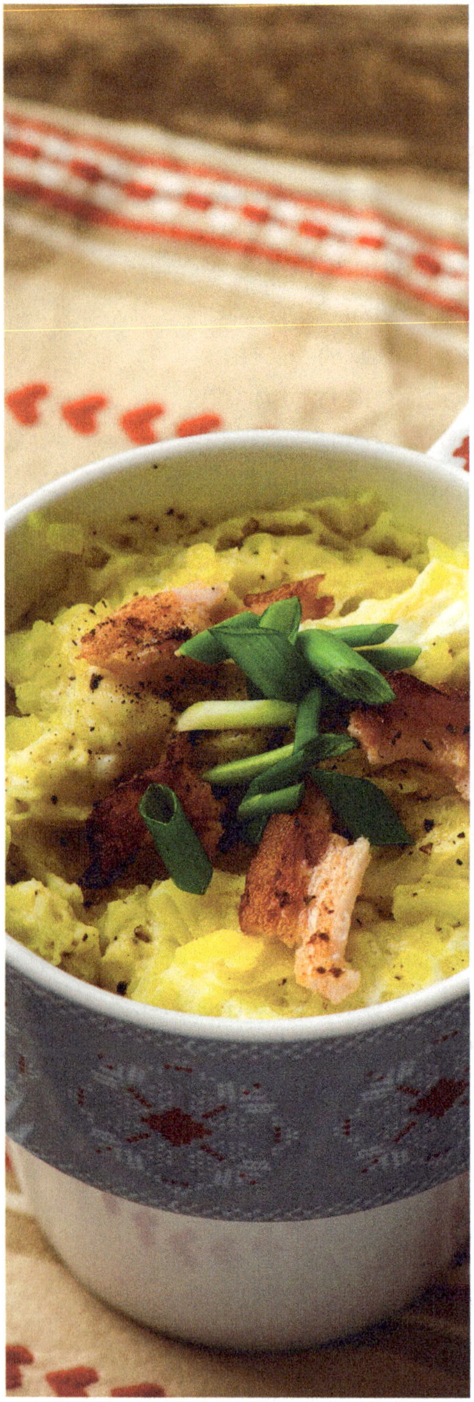

OMELET IN A MUG

Ingredients:

- 1 egg
- 2 tablespoons shredded cheese (cheddar, Swiss, pepper jack, etc.)
- 2 tablespoons diced ham, bacon, or sausage
- Salt (optional) and black pepper (optional) to taste

Instructions:

1. In a coffee mug, whisk together egg, cheese, ham, bacon, or sausage, salt (optional), and black pepper (optional).
2. Microwave on high for 1 minute. Stir and then microwave for an additional 30 seconds, or until omelet is cooked through. Serve immediately!

Serving Size: 1 omelet
Calories: 380

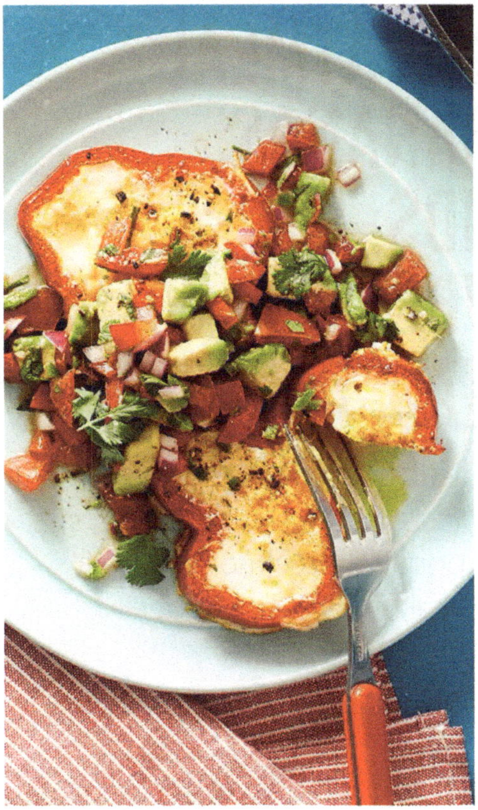

"EGG IN A HOLE" PEPPERS WITH AVOCADO SALSA

Ingredients:

- 2 large bell peppers, halved and seeded
- 4 eggs
- Salt (optional) and black pepper (optional) to taste

For the avocado salsa:

- 1 avocado, diced
- 1/4 cup diced tomatoes
- 1/4 cup diced onion
- 1 tablespoon chopped fresh cilantro
- Juice of 1 lime

Instructions:

1. Preheat oven to 350 degrees F.
2. Place bell pepper halves on a greased baking sheet. Crack an egg into the center of each pepper half. Season with salt (optional) and black pepper (optional).
3. Bake for 20-25 minutes, or until yolks are firm and whites are cooked through.
4. While peppers are cooking, prepare the avocado salsa by mixing together all ingredients in a small bowl.
5. Serve egg in a hole peppers with avocado salsa immediately!

Serving Size: 1 pepper half with 1/4 of the salsa
Calories: 310

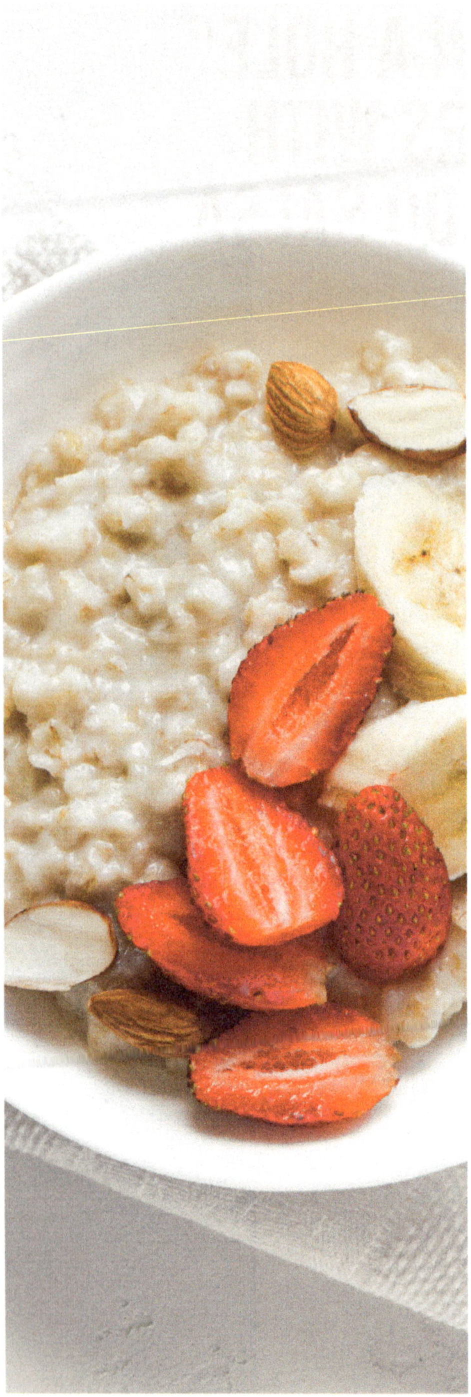

SAVORY OATMEAL WITH BANANAS, ALMONDS, & STRAWBERRIES WITH BANANAS, ALMONDS, & STRAWBERRIES

Ingredients:

- 1/2 cup quick-cooking oats
- 1/4 cup diced strawberries
- 1/4 cup diced bananas
- 2 tablespoons sliced almonds
- Salt (optional) and black pepper (optional) to taste

Instructions:

1. In a small bowl, mix together oats, strawberries, bananas, salt (optional), and almonds.
2. Microwave on high for 1-2 minutes, or until oatmeal is cooked through. Serve immediately!

Serving Size: 1 bowl of oatmeal
Calories: 350

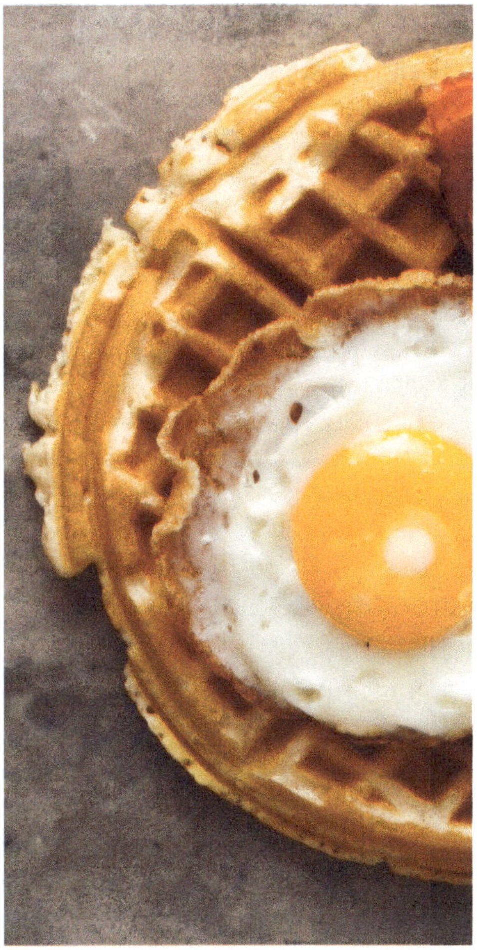

SOUTHWESTERN WAFFLE WITH FRIED EGG

Ingredients:

- 1/2 cup whole wheat flour
- 1/2 cup cornmeal
- 1 tablespoon Stevia
- 1 teaspoon baking powder
- 1/4 teaspoon salt (optional)
- 1 egg, beaten
- 1 cup milk (1% dairy, almond, or soy)
- 2 tablespoons oil (vegetable, canola, etc.)

Toppings:

- Fried egg
- Diced avocado
- Diced tomatoes
- Salsa

Instructions:

1. In a large bowl, mix together flour, cornmeal, Stevia, baking powder, and salt (optional).
2. In a separate bowl, whisk together egg, milk, and oil. Stir into the dry ingredients until just combined.
3. Cook waffles according to your waffle iron's instructions. Top with a fried egg, diced avocado, diced tomatoes, and salsa. Serve immediately!

Serving Size: 1 waffle with toppings
Calories: 430

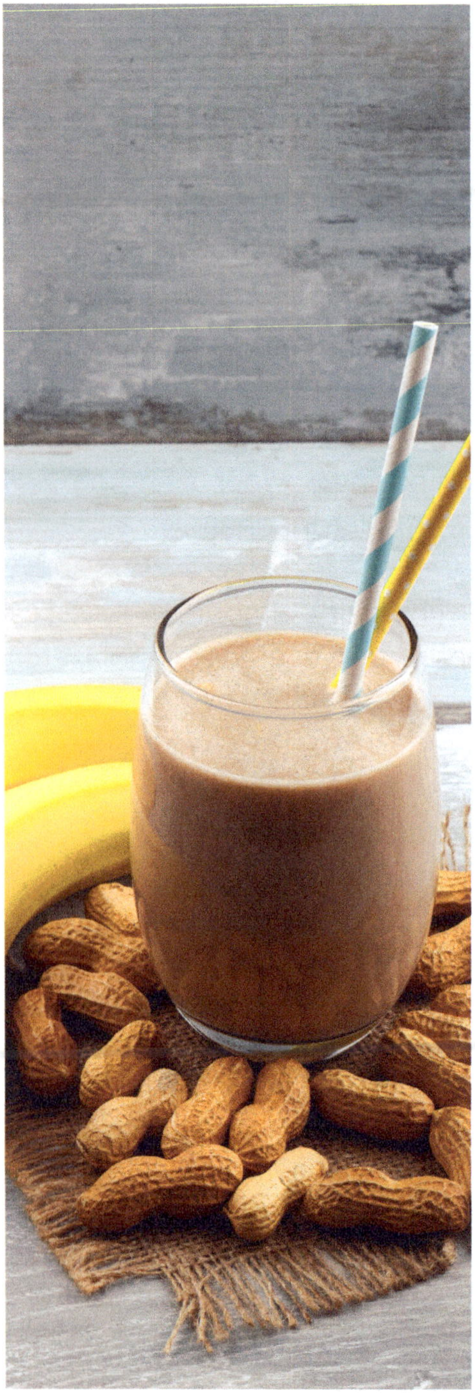

BANANA PEANUT BUTTER BREAKFAST SMOOTHIE

Ingredients:

- 1 large banana, sliced and frozen
- 1 cup milk (1% dairy, almond, or soy)
- 2 tablespoons peanut butter

Instructions:

1. In a blender, combine banana, milk, peanut butter, and ice (optional). Blend until smooth.
2. Pour into a glass and enjoy immediately!

Serving Size: 1 smoothie
Calories: 440

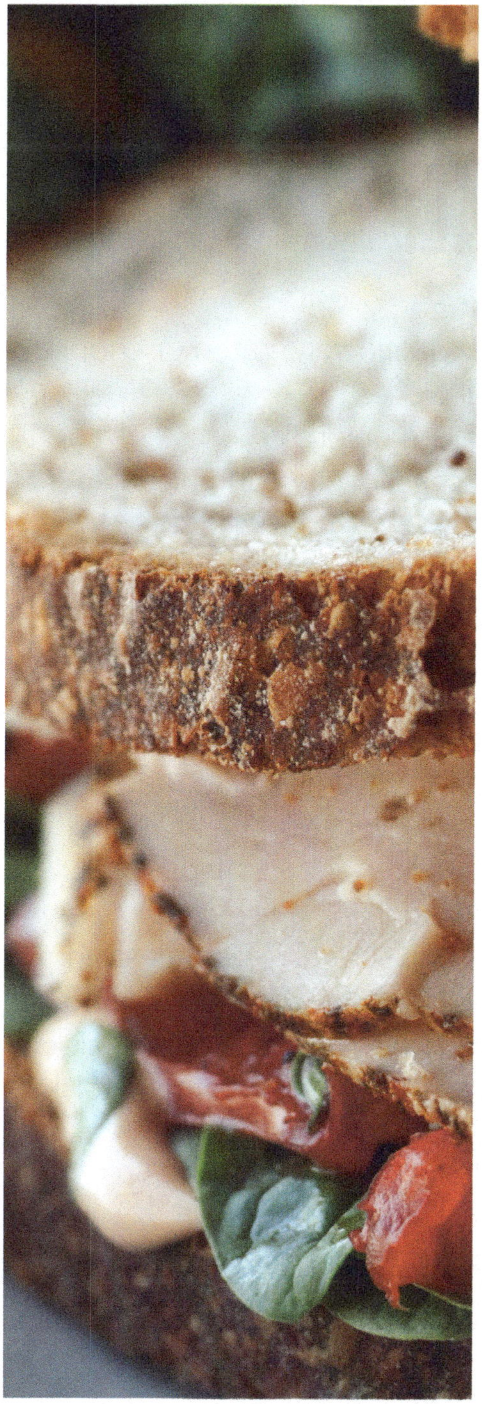

TURKEY, APPLE, AND CHEDDAR SANDWICH

Ingredients:

- 2 slices whole wheat bread
- 2 tablespoons cranberry sauce
- 1/4 cup thinly sliced turkey
- 1 small apple, thinly sliced
- 1 ounce cheddar cheese, shredded or sliced

Instructions:

1. Spread cranberry sauce on one slice of bread. Top with turkey, apple slices, and cheddar cheese. Top with remaining slice of bread.
2. Enjoy as is or grill in a panini press for 3-5 minutes, or until bread is toasted and cheese is melted. Serve immediately!

Serving Size: 1 sandwich
Calories: 430

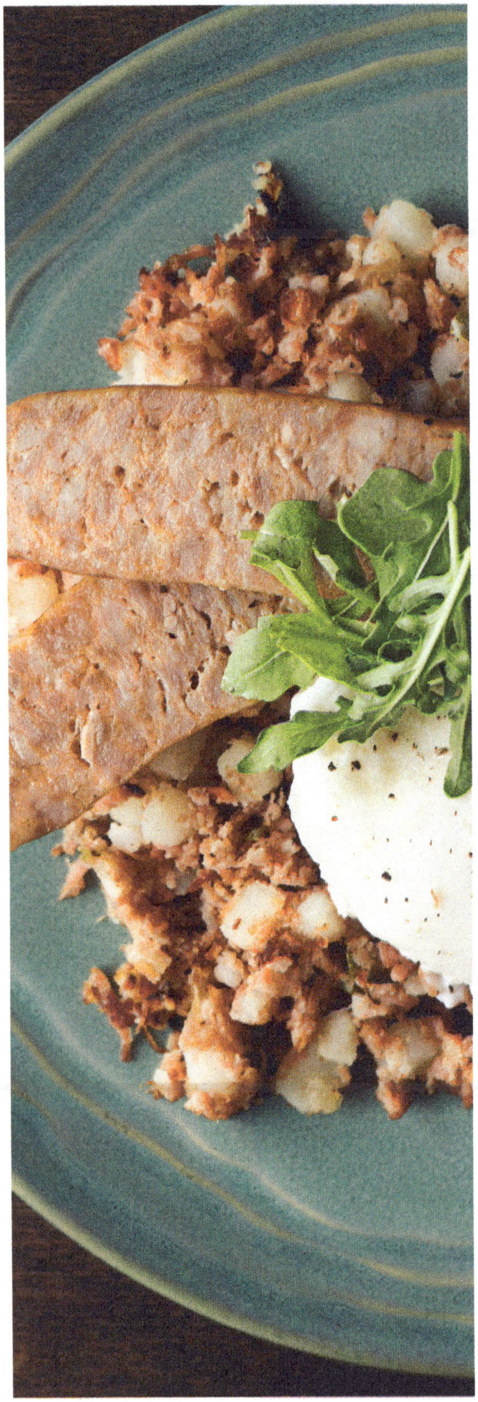

CAULIFLOWER HASH WITH SAUSAGE, EGGS, AND KALE

Ingredients:

- 1/2 head cauliflower, grated or chopped into small pieces
- 1/4 cup diced onion
- 1 link sausage, cooked and diced
- 2 eggs
- 1/4 cup chopped kale
- Salt (optional) and black pepper (optional) to taste

Instructions:

1. In a large skillet, cook cauliflower, onion, and sausage over medium heat until cauliflower is tender and sausage is cooked through.
2. Add eggs and scramble until desired doneness is reached. Stir in kale and season with salt (optional) and black pepper (optional). Serve immediately!

Serving Size: 1 portion of hash
Calories: 360

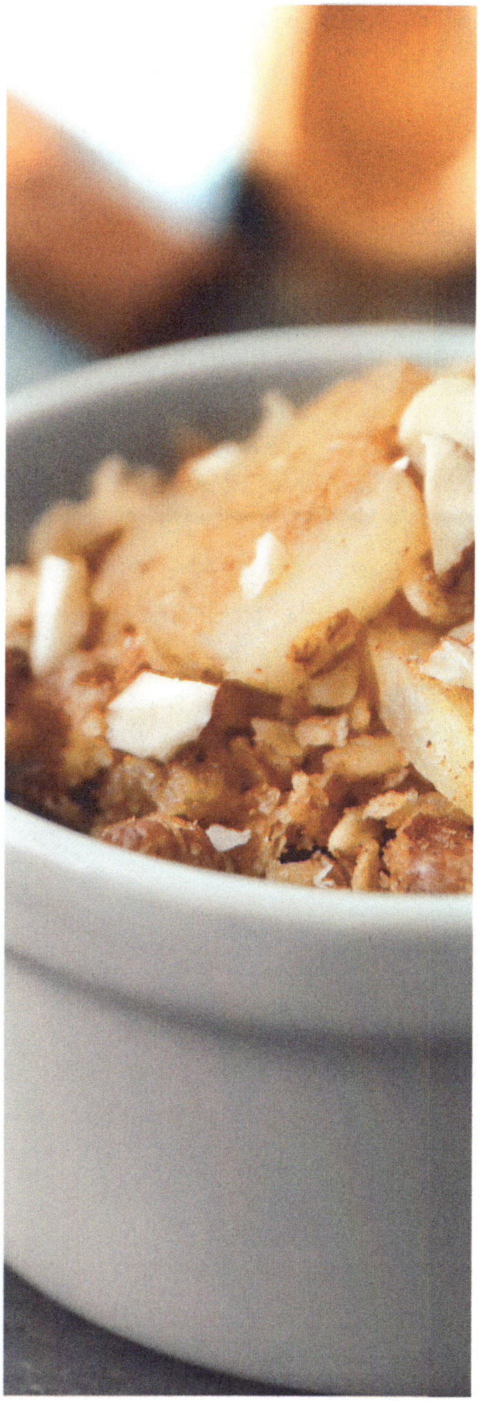

APPLE CRISP OATMEAL BOWL

Ingredients:

- 1/2 cup quick-cooking oats
- 1 small apple, diced
- 1 tablespoon Stevia
- 1/4 teaspoon cinnamon

Instructions:

1. In a small bowl, mix together oats, apple, Stevia, and cinnamon.
2. Microwave on high for 1-2 minutes, or until oatmeal is cooked through. Serve immediately!

Serving Size: 1 bowl of oatmeal
Calories: 340

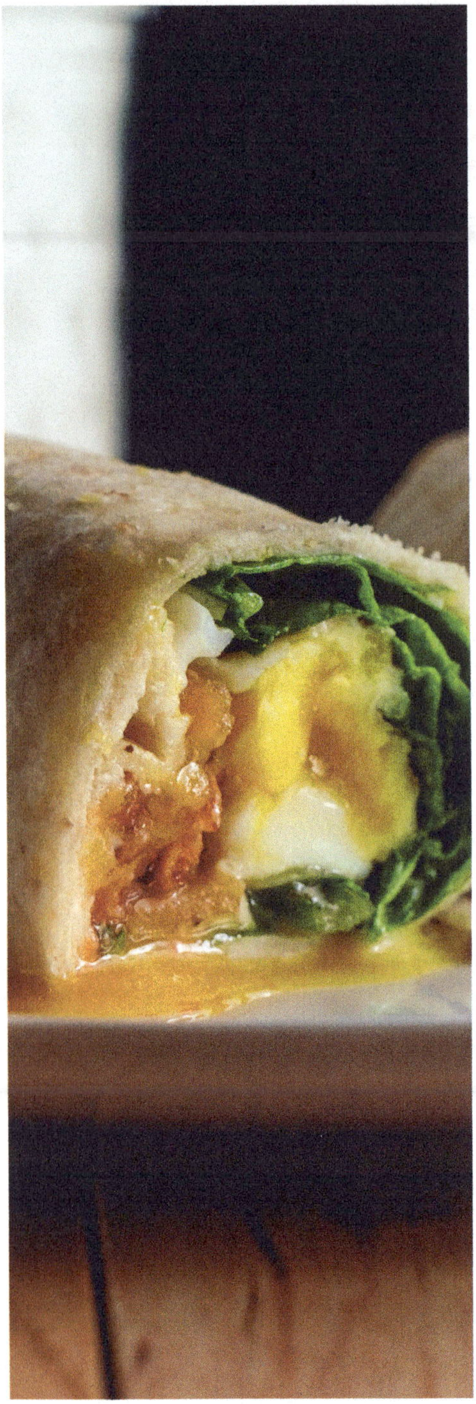

SPICY EGG WRAP

Ingredients:

- 1 whole wheat tortilla wrap
- 1 egg, beaten
- 1/4 cup shredded cheddar cheese (optional)
- 1 tablespoon diced green chilies

Instructions:

1. In a small skillet, cook egg over easy or to desired doneness.
2. Place cooked egg in the center of the tortilla wrap. Top with cheddar cheese (optional) and green chilies.
3. Roll up the wrap and enjoy immediately!

Serving Size: 1 wrap
Calories: 350

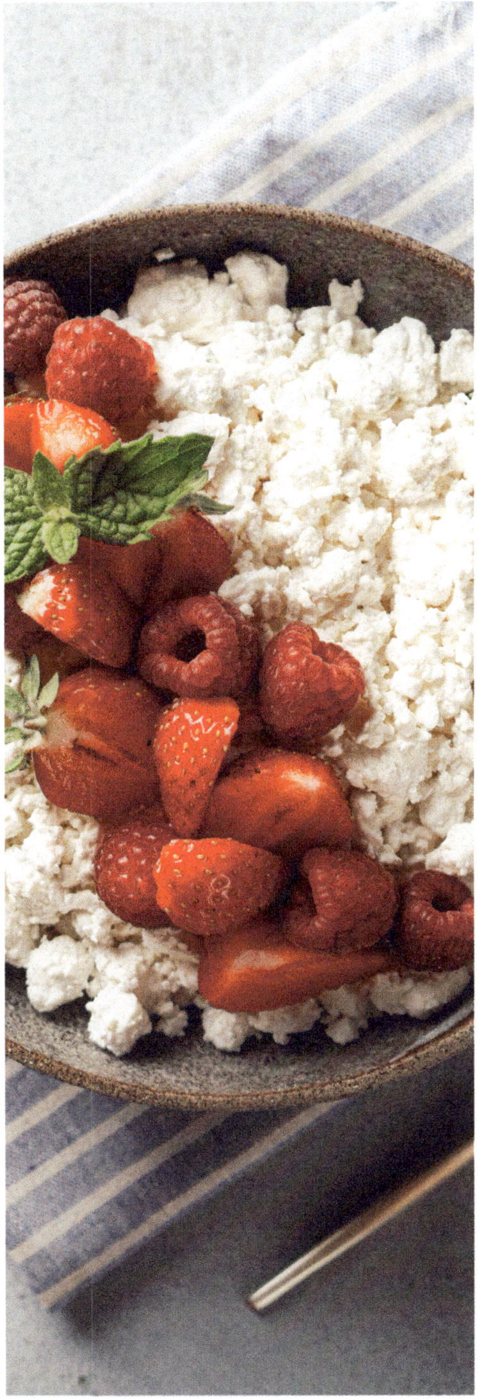

COTTAGE CHEESE WITH NUTS AND FRUIT

Ingredients:

- 1/2 cup cottage cheese
- 1/4 cup chopped nuts (almonds, peanuts, walnuts, etc.)
- 1/4 cup diced fruit (apple, pear, berries, etc.)

Instructions:

1. In a small bowl, mix together cottage cheese, nuts, and fruit. Serve immediately!

Serving Size: 1 portion of cottage cheese mixture
Calories: 360

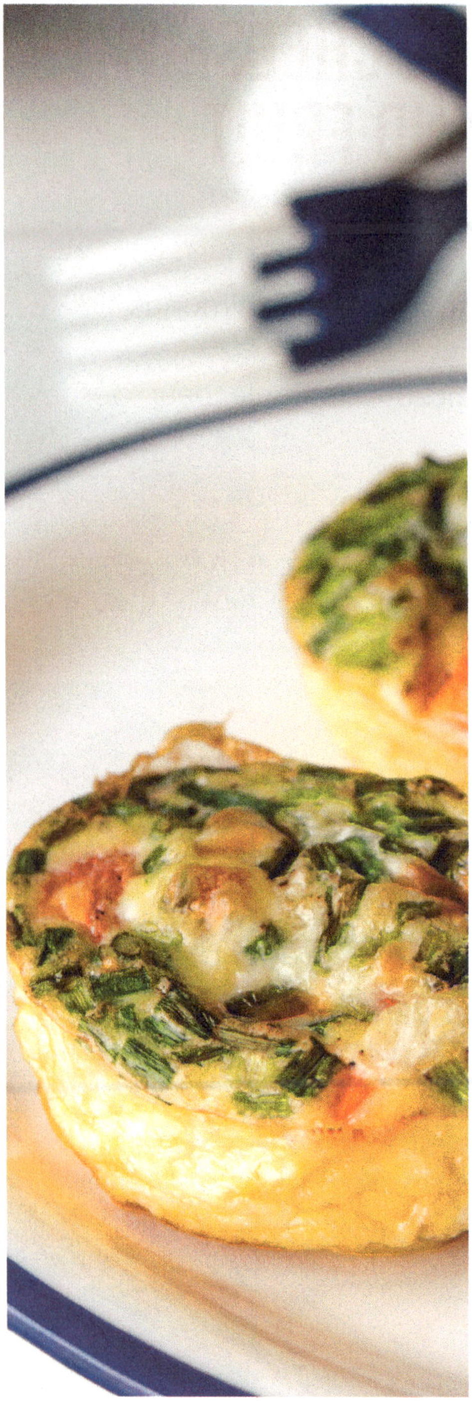

SPINACH EGG WHITE MUFFINS

Ingredients:

- 1/2 cup egg whites
- 1/4 cup diced onion
- 1/4 cup chopped spinach
- 1/4 cup shredded cheddar cheese (optional)

Instructions:

1. Preheat oven to 350 degrees Fahrenheit. Grease a muffin tin or line with paper liners.
2. In a large bowl, whisk together egg whites, onion, spinach, and cheddar cheese (optional).
3. Pour mixture into the prepared muffin tin, filling each muffin cup about 3/4 full. Bake for 15-20 minutes, or until eggs are cooked through. Serve immediately!

Serving Size: 1 egg muffin
Calories: 80

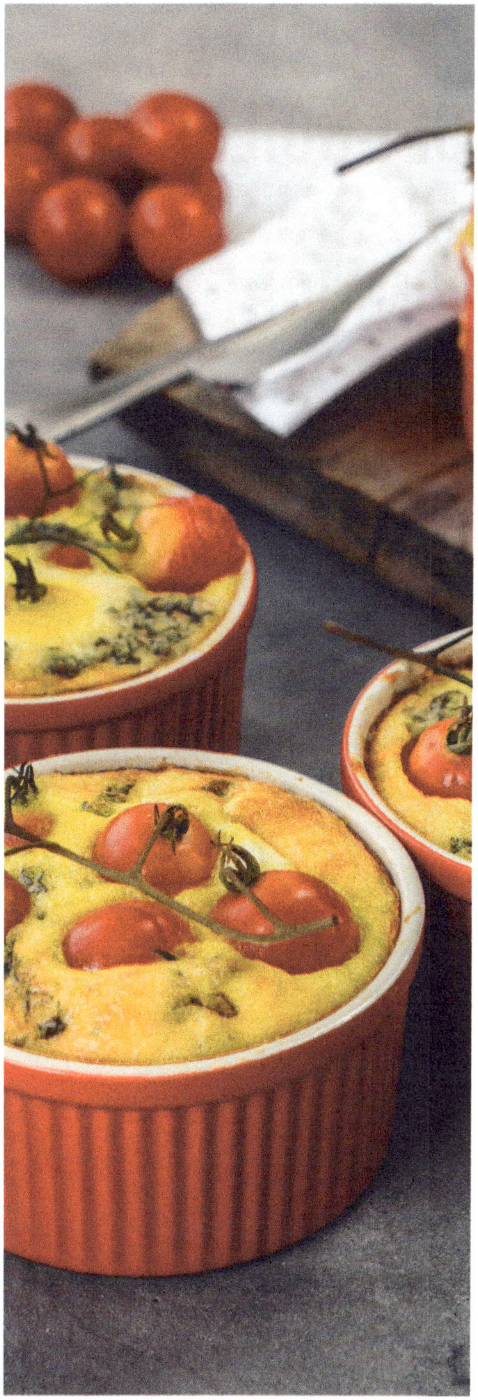

TOMATO-PARMESAN MINI QUICHES

Ingredients:

- 1/4 cup shredded Parmesan cheese
- 1/4 cups diced tomatoes
- 6 eggs

Instructions:

1. Preheat oven to 350 degrees Fahrenheit. Grease a muffin tin or line with paper liners.
2. In a large bowl, whisk together Parmesan cheese, tomatoes, and eggs.
3. Pour mixture into the prepared muffin tin, filling each muffin cup about 3/4 full. Bake for 15-20 minutes, or until eggs are cooked through. Serve immediately!

Serving Size: 1 quiche
Calories: 90

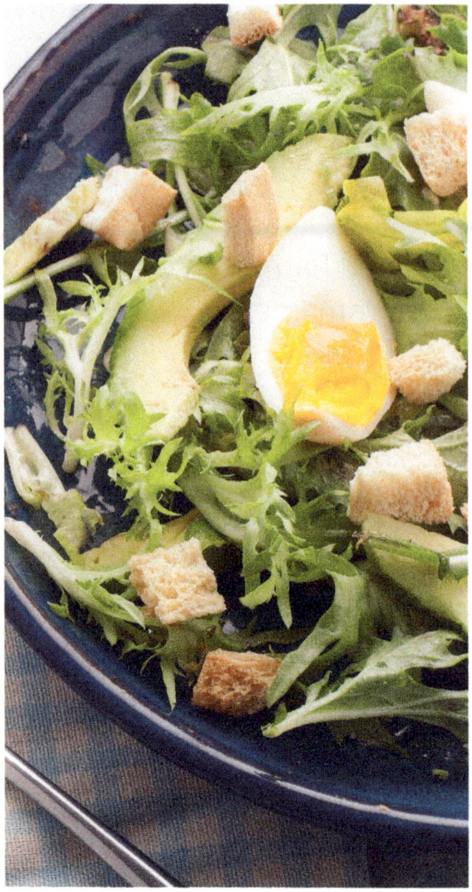

BREAKFAST SALAD WITH SOFT-BOILED EGGS AND SALSA VERDE VINAIGRETTE

Ingredients:

- 2 eggs
- 1 head romaine lettuce, chopped
- 1/4 cup diced tomatoes
- 1/4 cup shredded cheddar cheese (optional)
- 2 tablespoons salsa verde vinaigrette

For the salsa verde vinaigrette:

- 1/4 cup salsa verde
- 1 tablespoon olive oil
- 1 tablespoon red wine vinegar

Instructions:

1. In a small pot, bring water to a boil. Carefully add eggs and cook for 6 minutes. Remove from heat and let eggs sit in the hot water for an additional 2 minutes. Carefully remove eggs and place in ice water.
2. In a large bowl, mix together chopped lettuce, diced tomatoes, cheddar cheese (optional), and salsa verde vinaigrette.
3. Place eggs on top of the salad. Serve immediately!

Serving Size: 1 salad
Calories: 280

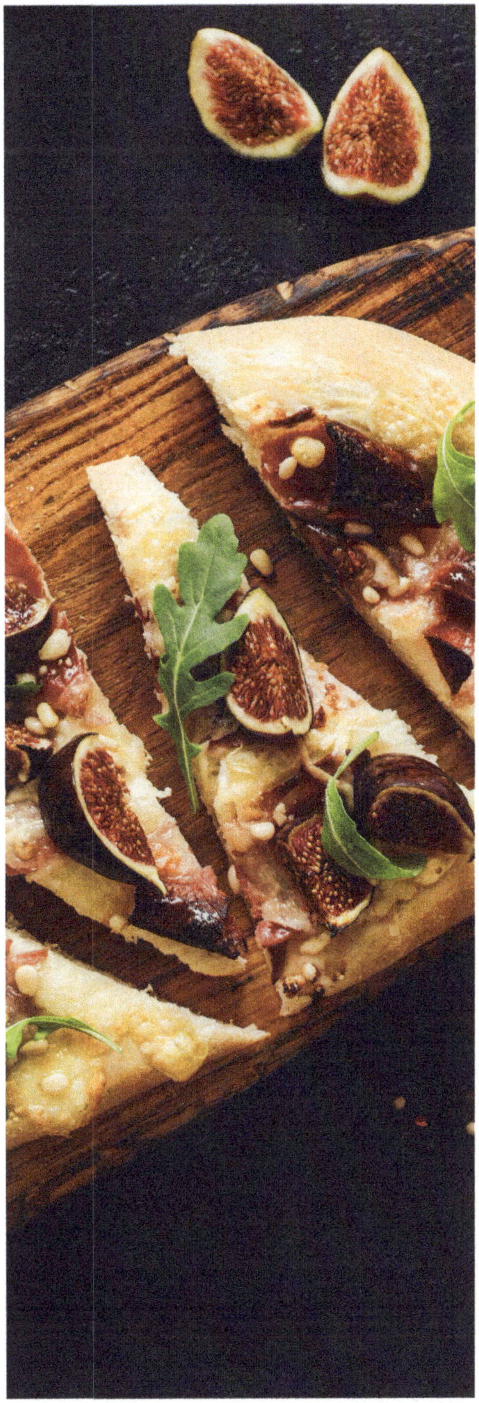

PEANUT BUTTER AND FIG ROASTED FLATBREAD

Ingredients:

- 1 whole wheat tortilla
- 2 tablespoons peanut butter
- 1/4 cup diced figs

Instructions:

1. Preheat oven to 350 degrees Fahrenheit.
2. Spread peanut butter on the tortilla, and then top with diced figs. Place the flatbread on a baking sheet and bake for 10-15 minutes, or until tortilla is crispy. Serve immediately!

Serving Size: 1 flatbread
Calories: 340

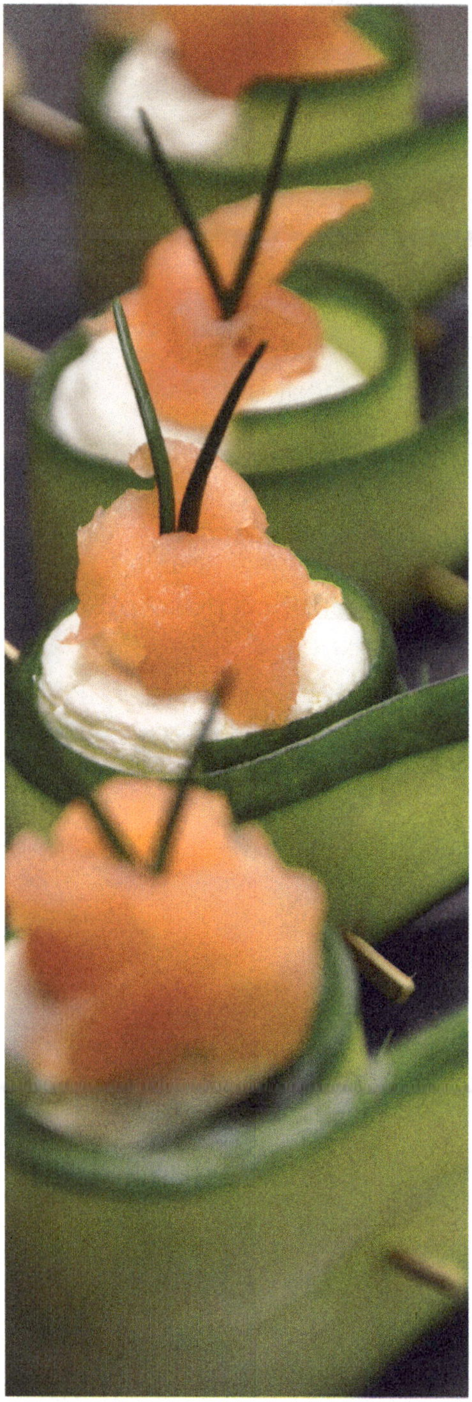

SALMON CUCUMBER ROLL-UPS

Ingredients:

- 4 ounces smoked salmon
- 1/2 cucumber, sliced into thin strips

Instructions:

1. Lay out a piece of salmon. Top with cucumber strips, and then roll up the salmon. Repeat with remaining salmon and cucumber slices. Serve immediately!

Serving Size: 2 roll-ups
Calories: 190

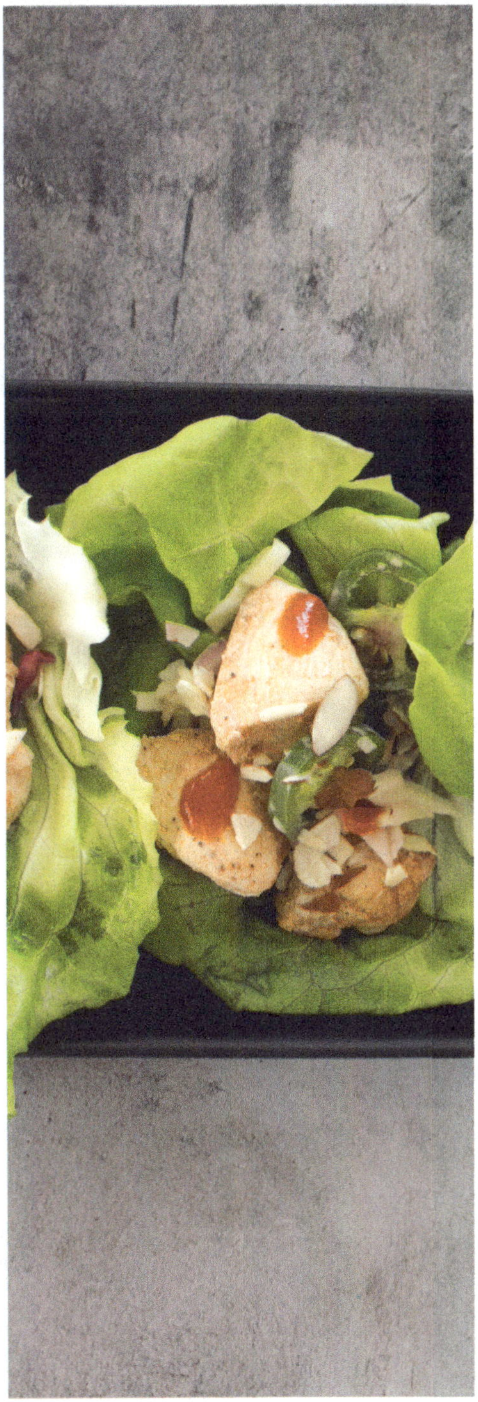

CURRIED CHICKEN SALAD LETTUCE WRAPS

Ingredients:

- 1/2 cup chopped cooked chicken
- 1/4 cup diced grapes
- 1 tablespoon diced celery
- 1 tablespoon diced onion
- 1 teaspoon curry powder

Instructions:

1. In a small bowl, mix together chopped chicken, grapes, celery, onion, and curry powder.
2. Serve mixture on lettuce leaves and enjoy immediately!

Serving Size: 1 lettuce wrap
Calories: 210

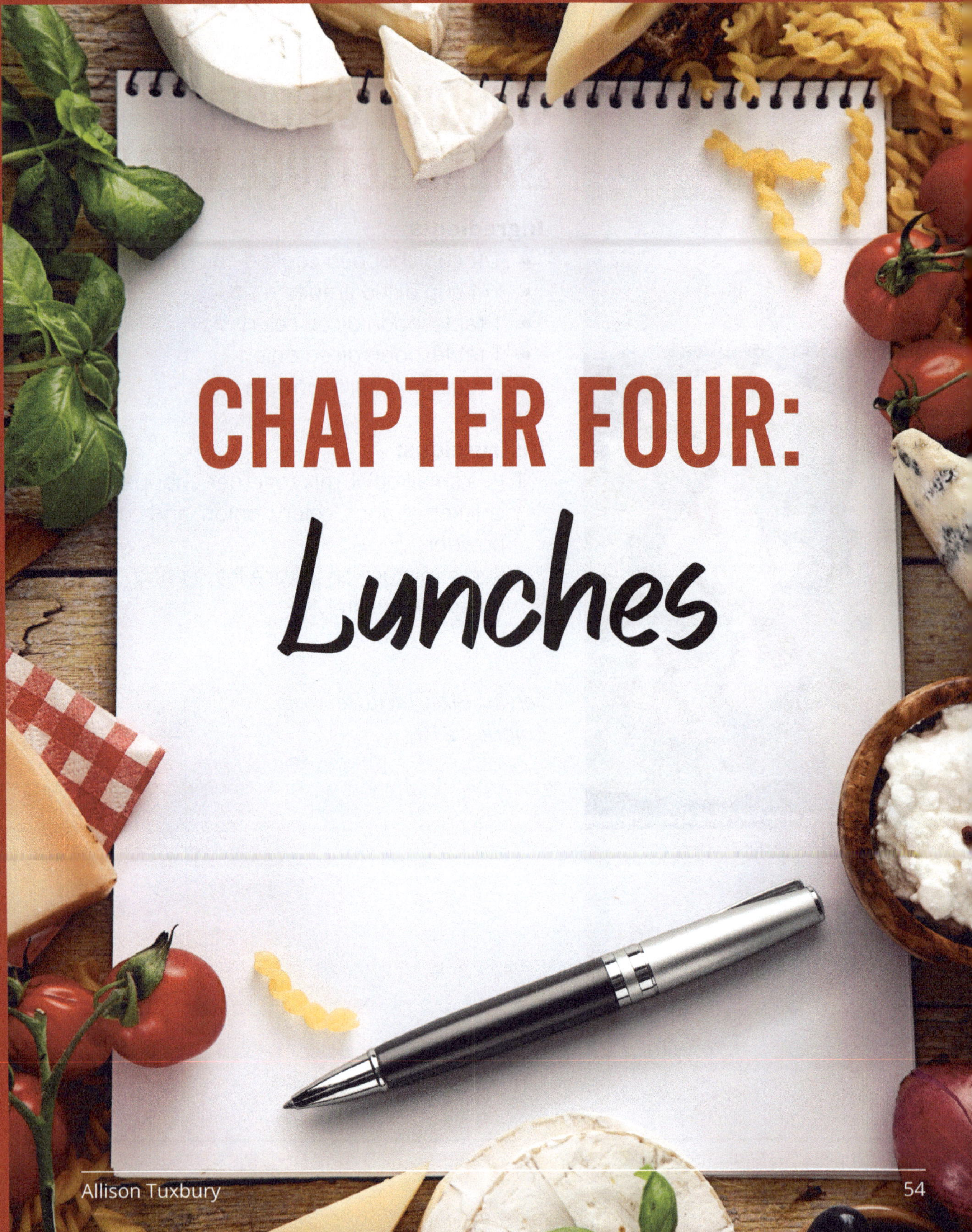

CHAPTER FOUR: Lunches

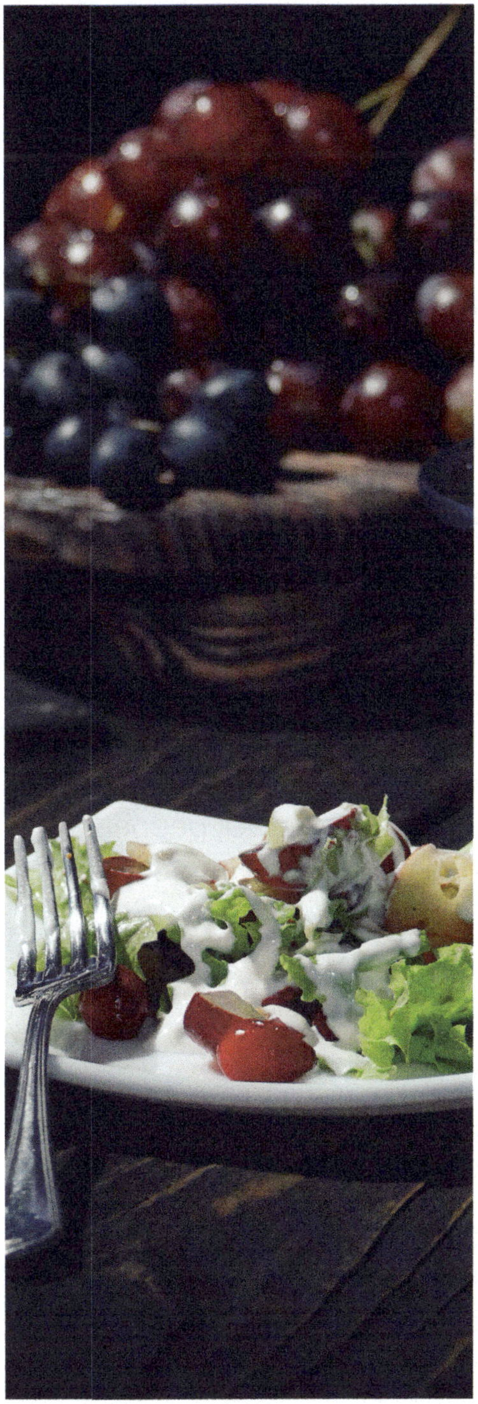

GREEK YOGURT CHICKEN SALAD (WRAP) WITH GRAPES

Ingredients:

- 1/2 cup diced cooked chicken breast
- 1/4 cup diced celery
- 1/4 cup grapes, halved
- 3 tablespoons plain Greek yogurt
- 1 tablespoon mayonnaise
- 1 teaspoon Dijon mustard
- Salt (optional) and black pepper (optional) to taste
- 1 whole wheat tortilla wrap (optional)

Instructions:

1. In a small bowl, mix together chicken, celery, grapes, Greek yogurt, mayonnaise, and Dijon mustard. Season with salt and black pepper (optional) to taste.
2. (Optional) Spread mixture evenly on tortilla wrap and roll up. Serve immediately!

Serving Size: 1 wrap
Calories: 420

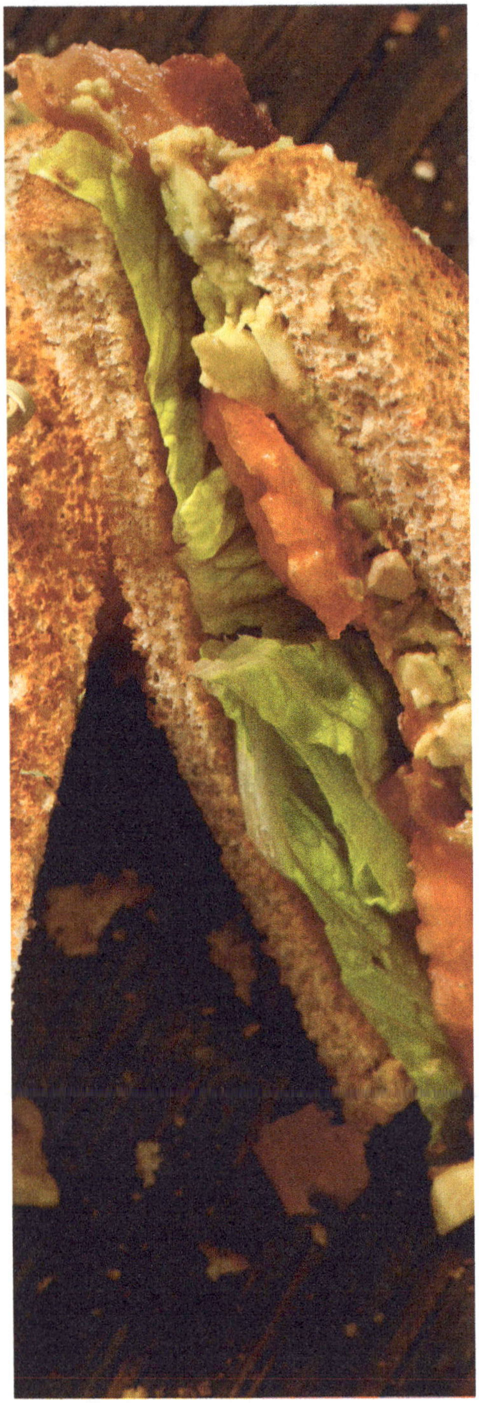

TURKEY AVOCADO BLT SANDWICH ON WHOLE WHEAT BREAD

Ingredients:

- 4 slices whole wheat bread, toasted
- 3 tablespoons mayonnaise
- 1 avocado, diced
- 8 slices turkey bacon, cooked
- 1 tomato, sliced
- Salt (optional) and black pepper (optional) to taste

Instructions:

1. Spread mayonnaise on toast slices. Top with avocado, turkey bacon, and tomato. Season with salt and black pepper (optional) to taste. Serve immediately!

Serving Size: 1 sandwich
Calories: 480

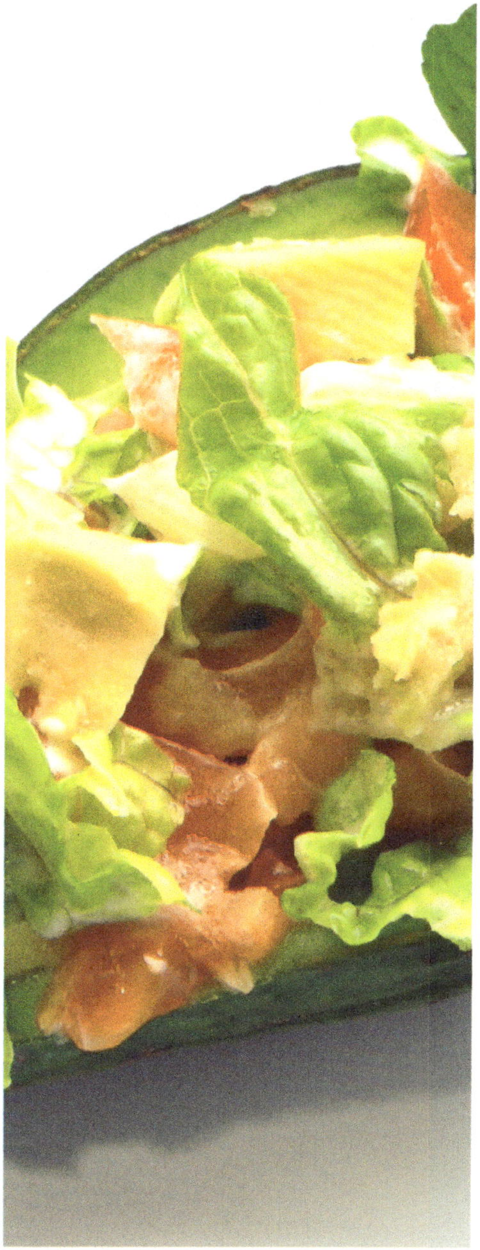

SALMON-STUFFED AVOCADOS WITH GOAT CHEESE

Ingredients:

- 2 avocados, halved and pitted
- 1/4 cup diced cooked salmon
- 1 tablespoon plain Greek yogurt
- 1 tablespoon finely diced red onion
- 1 clove garlic, minced
- 1 teaspoon lemon juice
- Salt (optional) and black pepper (optional) to taste
- 2 tablespoons goat cheese

Instructions:

1. In a medium bowl, mix together salmon, Greek yogurt, red onion, garlic, and lemon juice. Season with salt and black pepper (optional) to taste.
2. Spoon mixture evenly into avocado halves. Top with goat cheese. Serve immediately!

Serving Size: 1 stuffed avocado half
Calories: 290

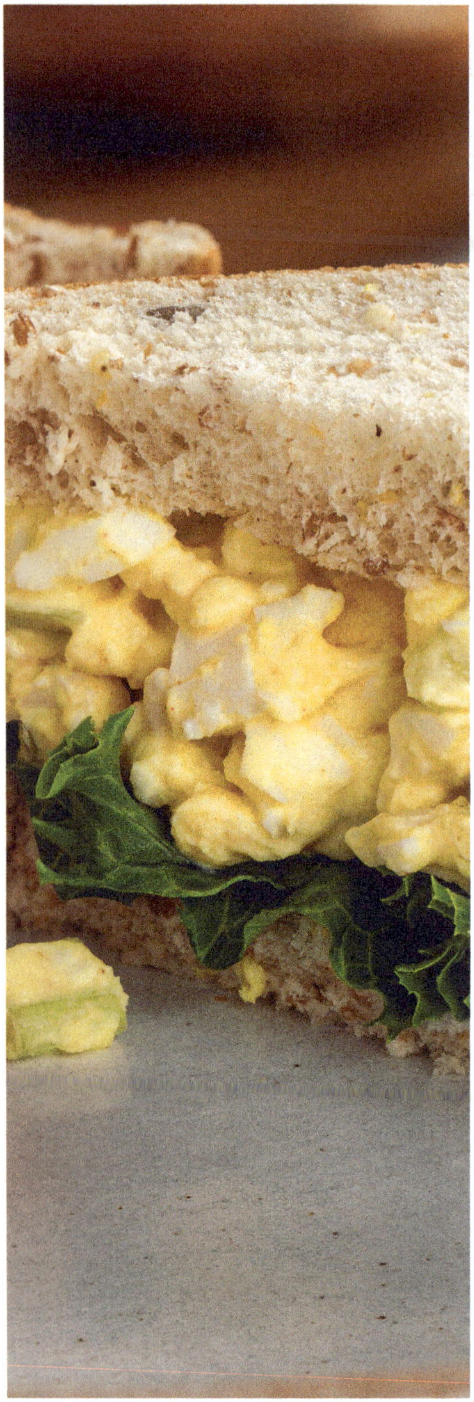

EGG SALAD SANDWICH ON WHOLE WHEAT BREAD

Ingredients:

- 1/4 cup diced celery
- 3 tablespoons diced red onion
- 6 hard-boiled eggs, diced
- 1/4 cup mayonnaise
- 1 tablespoon yellow mustard
- Salt (optional) and black pepper (optional) to taste
- 4 slices whole wheat bread, toasted

Instructions:

1. In a medium bowl, mix together celery, red onion, eggs, mayonnaise, and yellow mustard. Season with salt and black pepper (optional) to taste.
2. Spread mixture evenly on toast slices. Serve immediately!

Serving Size: 1 sandwich
Calories: 440

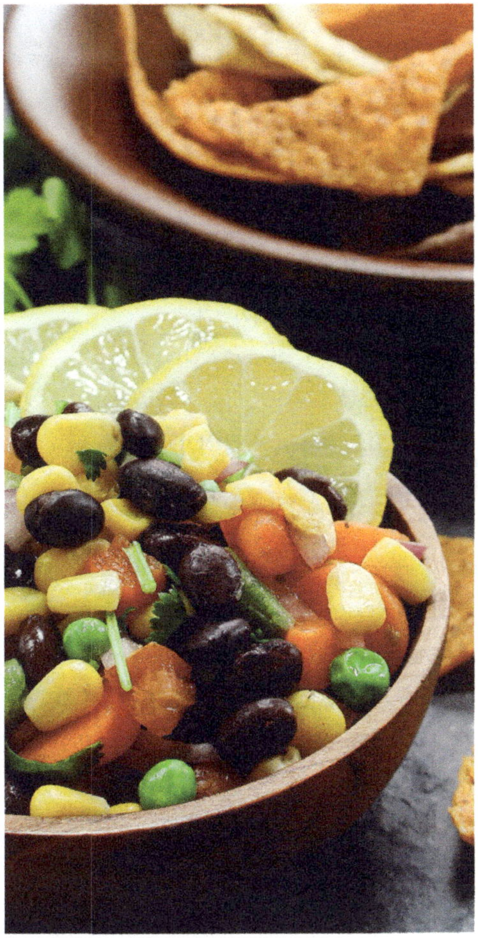

SOUTHWESTERN CHICKEN SALAD WITH BLACK BEANS AND CORN

Ingredients:

- 1/2 cup diced cooked chicken breast
- 1/4 cup black beans
- 1/4 cup corn kernels
- 3 tablespoons diced red onion
- 3 tablespoons diced green bell pepper
- 2 tablespoons diced jalapeño pepper
- 1 tablespoon finely chopped cilantro
- /4 cup plain Greek yogurt
- 1 clove garlic, minced
- Juice of 1 lime
- Salt (optional) and black pepper (optional) to taste

Instructions:

1. In a medium bowl, mix together chicken, black beans, corn, red onion, green bell pepper, jalapeño pepper, cilantro, Greek yogurt, garlic, and lime juice. Season with salt and black pepper (optional) to taste.
2. Serve immediately!

Serving Size: 1/2 cup
Calories: 140

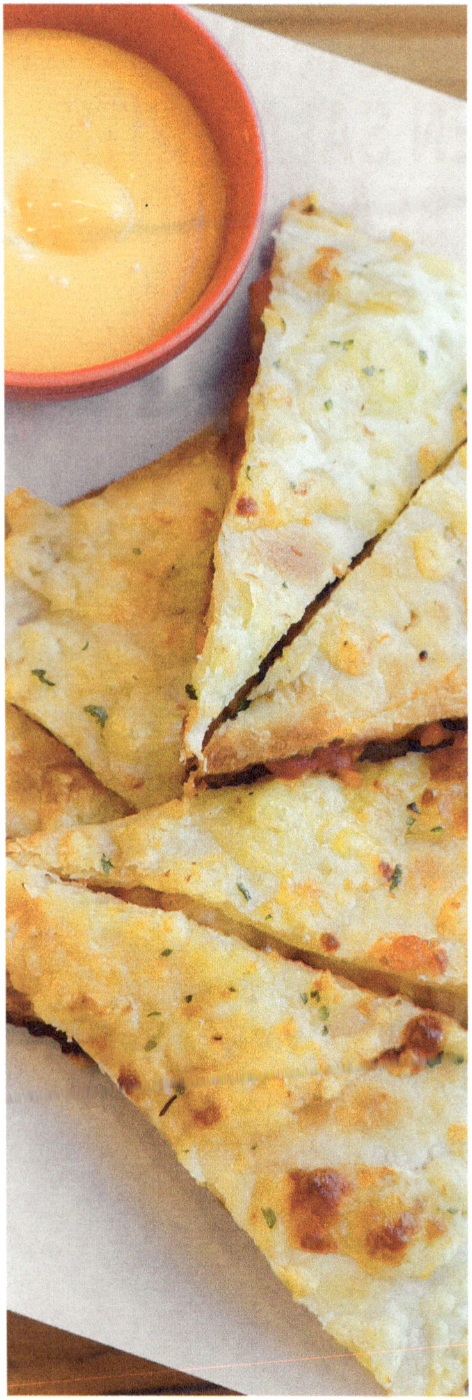

SWEET PEPPER-GREEN ONION QUESADILLAS

Ingredients:

- 4 whole wheat tortillas
- 1/4 cup diced sweet pepper
- 3 tablespoons diced green onion
- 1/2 cup shredded cheese
- Salt (optional) and black pepper (optional) to taste

Instructions:

1. Preheat grill to medium-high heat.
2. On a work surface, lay out 2 tortillas. Top each with sweet pepper, green onion, and cheese. Season with salt and black pepper (optional) to taste. Top each with remaining 2 tortillas.
3. Place quesadillas on grill and cook for 2-3 minutes per side, or until golden brown and cheese is melted. Cut each into 4 pieces and serve immediately!

Serving Size: 1 quesadilla
Calories: 320

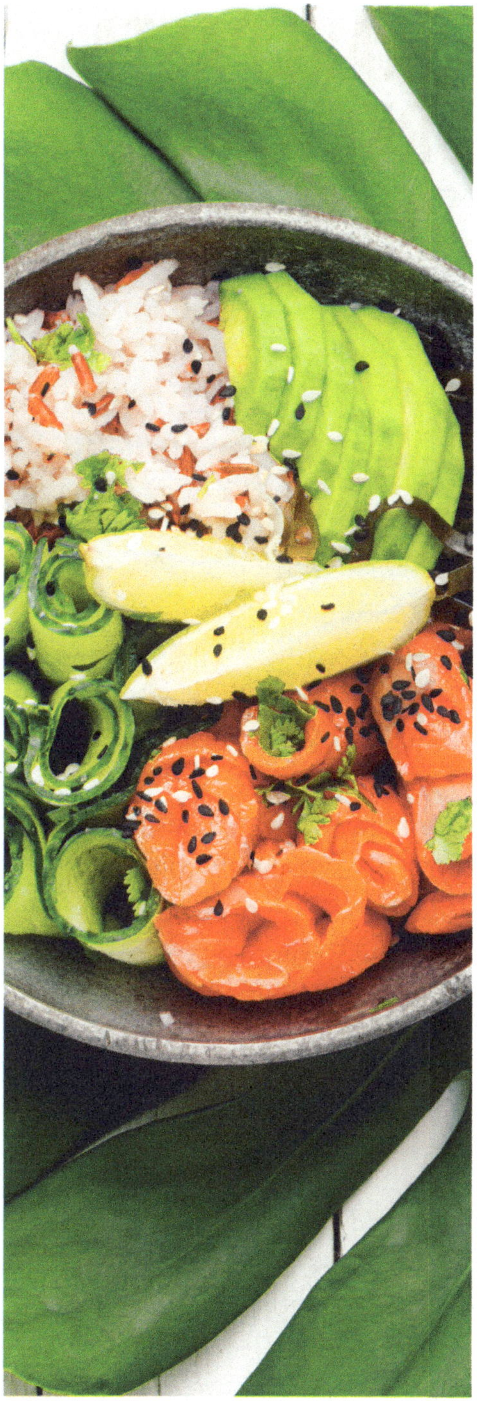

SALMON POKE BOWL WITH BROWN RICE

Ingredients:

- 1/2 cup cooked brown rice
- 1/4 cup diced cucumber
- 1/4 cup diced avocado
- 3 tablespoons diced red onion
- 1/4 cup shelled edamame
- 2 ounces salmon, diced
- 1 tablespoon finely chopped cilantro
- 1 teaspoon sesame oil (optional)

Instructions:

1. In a medium bowl, mix together brown rice, cucumber, avocado, red onion, edamame, salmon, cilantro, and sesame oil (optional).
2. Serve immediately!

Serving Size: 1 bowl
Calories: 400

WHOLE-GRAIN PASTA WITH TURKEY AND VEGGIES

Ingredients:

- 1/2 cup whole-grain pasta
- 1/4 cup diced cooked turkey
- 1/4 cup diced zucchini
- 1/4 cup diced yellow squash
- 3 tablespoons tomato sauce
- Salt (optional) and black pepper (optional) to taste

Instructions:

1. For the pasta, follow package directions.
2. In a medium saucepan, mix together turkey, zucchini, yellow squash, and tomato sauce. Season with salt and black pepper (optional) to taste. Cook over medium heat for 5 minutes, or until heated through.
3. Serve turkey mixture over cooked pasta. Serve immediately!

Serving Size: 1/2 cup
Calories: 290

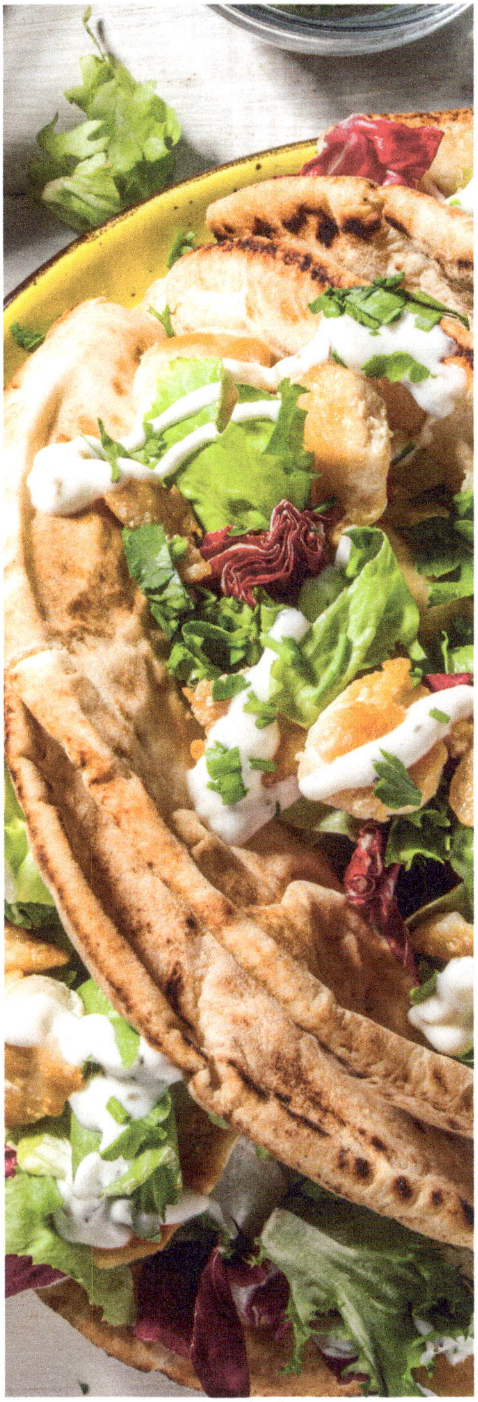

EGG AND BROCCOLI SLAW WRAP WITH TZATZIKI SAUCE

Ingredients:

- 1 whole wheat wrap
- 2 hard-boiled eggs, diced
- 1/4 cup broccoli slaw mix
- 3 tablespoons diced cucumber
- 2 tablespoons plain yogurt
- 1 clove garlic, minced
- Juice of 1/2 lemon
- Salt (optional) and black pepper (optional) to taste

Instructions:

1. In a small bowl, mix together cucumber, yogurt, garlic, and lemon juice. Season with salt and black pepper (optional) to taste. Set aside.
2. On a work surface, lay out the wrap. Top with eggs, broccoli slaw mix, and cucumber mixture. Roll up tightly and cut in half if desired. Serve immediately!

Serving Size: 1 wrap
Calories: 380

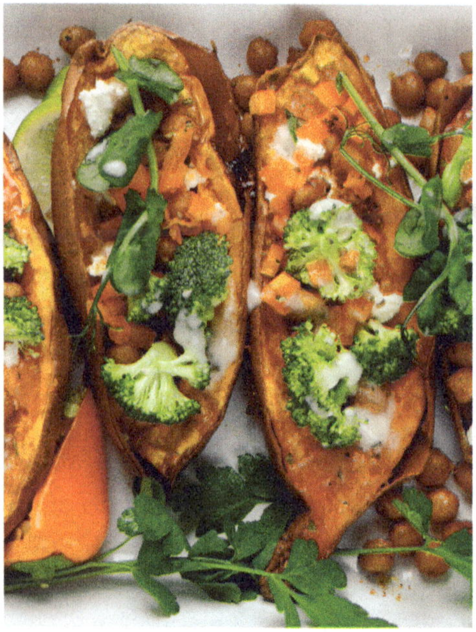

STUFFED SWEET POTATOES WITH SALSA AND BEANS

Ingredients:

- 2 large sweet potatoes
- 1/4 cup salsa
- 1/4 cup black beans
- 3 tablespoons diced green onion
- 1 ounce shredded cheese
- Salt (optional) and black pepper (optional) to taste

Instructions:

1. Preheat oven to 400 degrees F. Pierce sweet potatoes a few times with a fork and place on a baking sheet. Bake for 45 minutes, or until tender.
2. Remove from oven and let cool slightly. Cut each potato in half lengthwise and scoop out the flesh, leaving a 1/4-inch border.
3. In a medium bowl, mix together sweet potato flesh, salsa, black beans, green onion, and cheese. Season with salt and black pepper (optional) to taste.
4. Divide mixture evenly among sweet potato halves. Place on baking sheet and bake for 10-15 minutes, or until heated through. Serve Immediately!

Serving Size: 1 stuffed sweet potato half
Calories: 330

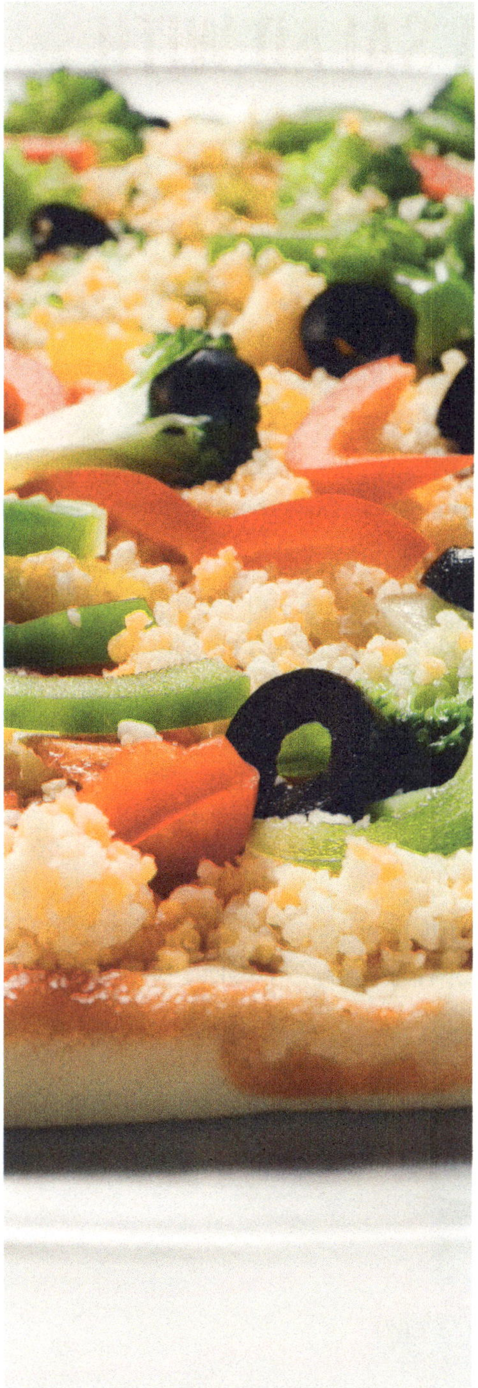

THIN-CRUST VEGETABLE PIZZA

Ingredients:

- 1/2 recipe thin-crust pizza dough
- 1/4 cup tomato sauce
- 1/4 cup shredded cheese
- 1/4 cup chopped broccoli
- 1/4 cup chopped cauliflower
- 1/4 cup diced red onion
- Salt (optional) and black pepper (optional) to taste

Instructions:

1. Preheat oven to 425 degrees F. Roll out pizza dough on a lightly floured surface and place on a baking sheet.
2. Spread tomato sauce evenly over dough. Sprinkle with cheese, broccoli, cauliflower, and red onion. Season with salt and black pepper (optional) to taste.
3. Bake for 15-20 minutes, or until crust is golden brown and cheese is melted. Serve immediately!

Serving Size: 1 slice
Calories: 230

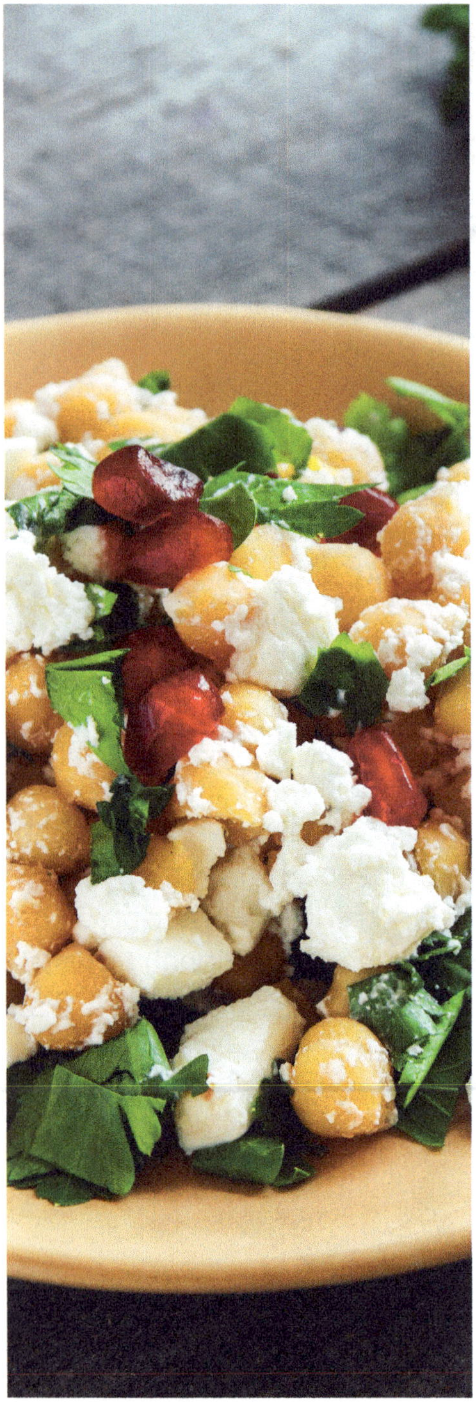

QUINOA SALAD WITH EDAMAME, CRANBERRIES, AND FETA

Ingredients:

- 1/2 cup cooked quinoa
- 1/2 cup cooked chickpeas (optional sub)
- 1/4 cup shelled edamame
- 1/4 cup dried cranberries
- 1/4 cup crumbled feta cheese
- 3 tablespoons diced red onion
- 1 tablespoon finely chopped parsley
- 1 tablespoon balsamic vinegar
- Salt (optional) and black pepper (optional) to taste

Instructions:

1. In a medium bowl, mix together quinoa, edamame, cranberries, feta cheese, red onion, parsley, and balsamic vinegar. Season with salt and black pepper (optional) to taste.
2. Serve at room temperature or chilled. Enjoy!

Serving Size: 1/2 cup
Calories: 220

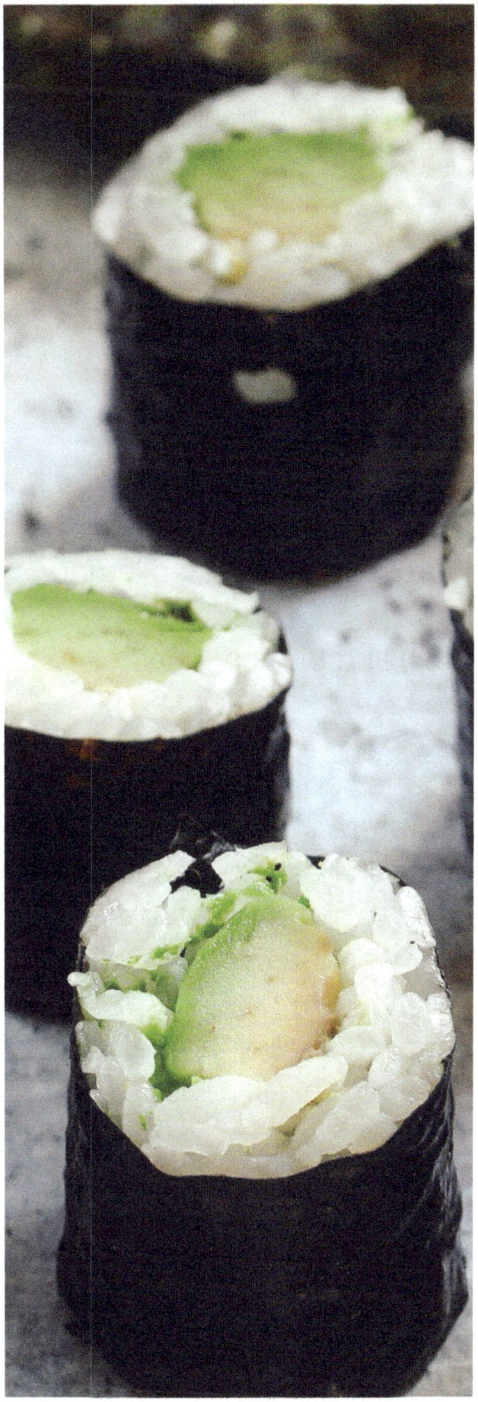

CUCUMBER, AVOCADO, AND RICE SUSHI ROLLS

Ingredients:

- 1/2 cup cooked rice
- 1/4 cucumber, peeled and seeded
- 1/4 avocado, diced
- 1 nori sheet
- Water, for sealing sushi rolls

Instructions:

1. Place the nori sheet on a bamboo sushi roller (or a clean work surface). Spread rice evenly over nori, leaving a 1-inch border at the bottom.
2. Place cucumber and avocado in a line down the center of the rice. Starting at the top, roll the sushi tightly until the nori is sealed.
3. Using a sharp knife, cut sushi into 8 pieces. Serve with soy sauce (optional) and wasabi (optional). Enjoy!

Serving Size: 2 sushi rolls (4 pieces each)
Calories: 190

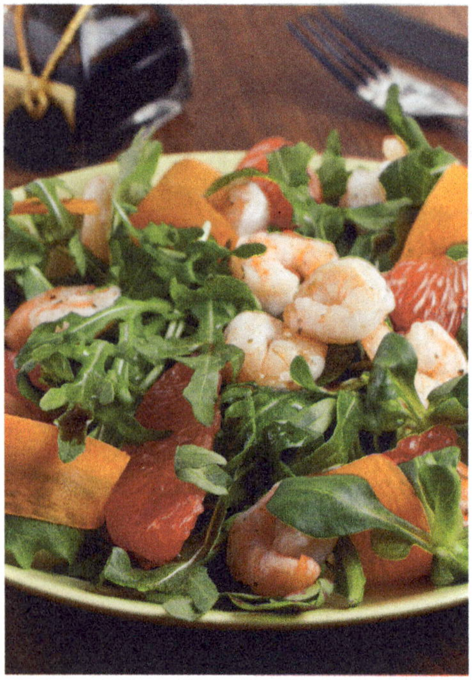

LEMON SHRIMP AND ORZO SALAD

Ingredients:

- 1/2 cup orzo
- 1/2 cup mixed greens (optional sub)
- 1/4 pound shrimp, peeled and deveined
- 1/4 cup diced English cucumber
- 1/4 cup diced red grapes
- 1/4 cup crumbled feta cheese
- 3 tablespoons chopped parsley
- 1 tablespoon freshly squeezed lemon juice
- Salt (optional) and black pepper (optional) to taste

Instructions:

1. For the orzo, bring a large pot of water to a boil and cook orzo according to package instructions. Drain and rinse with cold water.
2. For the shrimp, heat a large skillet over medium-high heat. Season shrimp with salt and black pepper (optional) to taste. Add to skillet and cook for 2-3 minutes per side, or until opaque. Remove from heat and chop into bite-sized pieces.
3. In a large bowl, mix together cooked orzo, shrimp, cucumber, grapes, feta cheese, parsley, and lemon juice. Season with salt and black pepper (optional) to taste.
4. Serve at room temperature or chilled. Enjoy!

Serving Size: 1/2 cup
Calories: 250

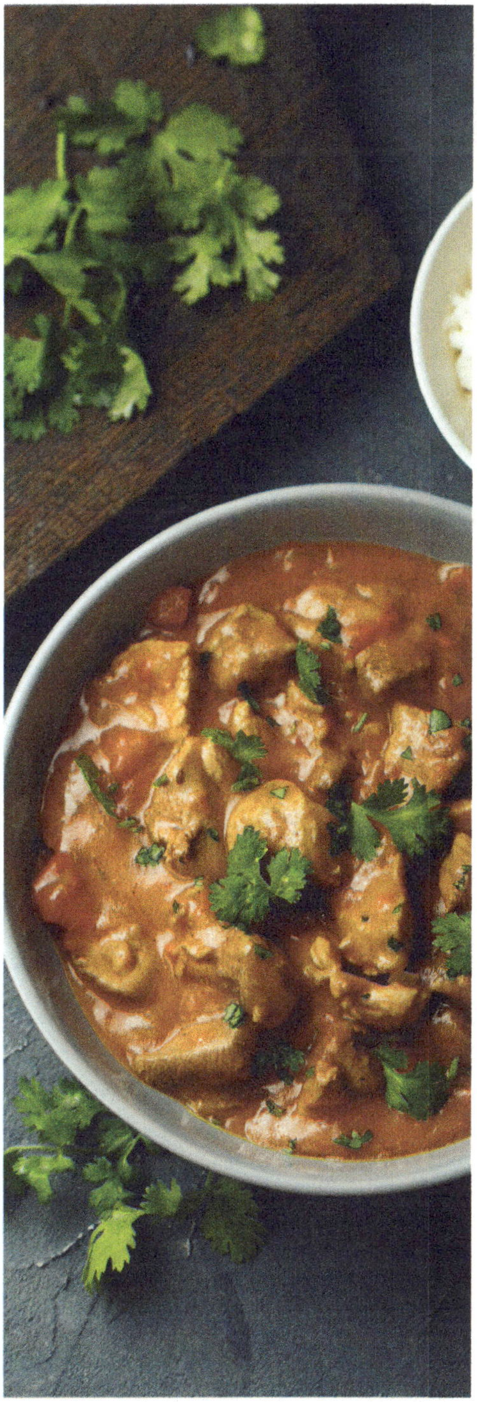

CURRIED CHICKEN SKILLET

Ingredients:

- 1/2 pound boneless, skinless chicken breasts, cut into bite-sized pieces
- 1 tablespoon olive oil
- 1 yellow onion, diced
- 2 cloves garlic, minced
- 1 tablespoon curry powder
- 1/4 teaspoon ground ginger
- Salt (optional) and black pepper (optional) to taste

Instructions:

1. Heat a large skillet over medium-high heat. Add chicken, olive oil, onion, garlic, curry powder, ginger, salt and black pepper (optional) to the skillet.
2. Cook for 6-8 minutes, or until chicken is cooked through and onion is softened. Serve immediately!

Serving Size: 1/2 cup
Calories: 260

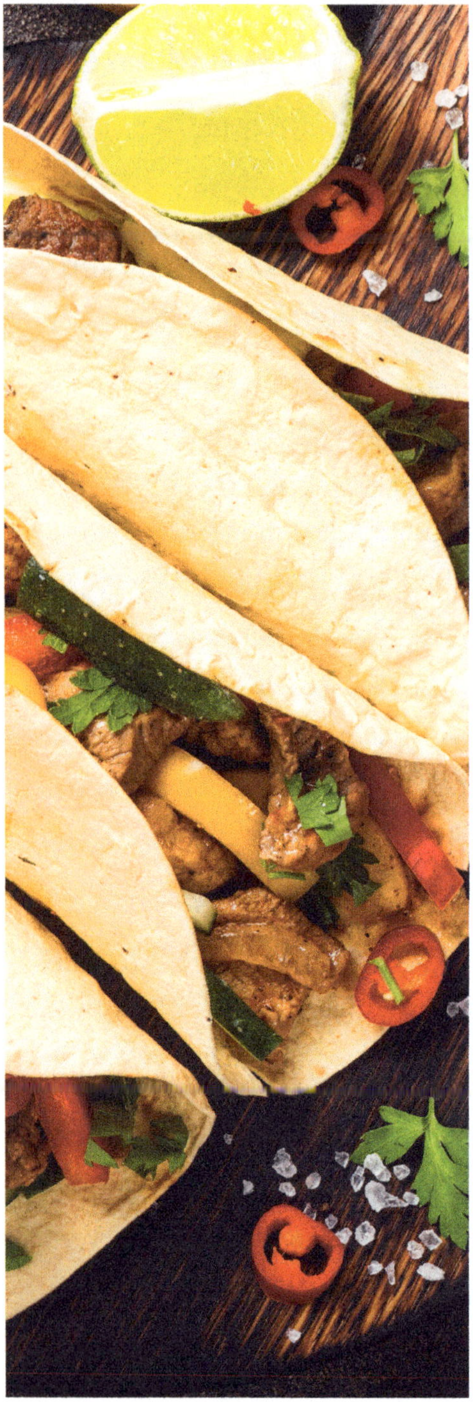

PRESSURE-COOKER PORK TACOS WITH MANGO SALSA

Ingredients:

- 1/2 pound pork loin, cut into 1-inch cubes
- 1 tablespoon olive oil
- 1 yellow onion, diced
- 2 cloves garlic, minced
- 1 tablespoon chili powder
- 1 teaspoon ground cumin
- Salt (optional) and black pepper (optional) to taste

For the mango salsa:

- 1 mango, peeled and diced
- 1/4 red onion, diced
- 1 small jalapeño pepper, seeded and diced
- 2 tablespoons chopped fresh cilantro leaves
- 1 tablespoon freshly squeezed lime juice

Instructions:

1. Add pork, olive oil, onion, garlic, chili powder, cumin, salt and black pepper (optional) to the pressure cooker. Cook according to manufacturer's instructions.
2. Meanwhile, in a medium bowl, mix together mango, red onion, jalapeño pepper, cilantro, and lime juice. Season with salt and black pepper (optional) to taste.
3. When pork is cooked through, remove from pressure cooker and let cool for 5 minutes. Using two forks, shred the pork.
4. Serve shredded pork on soft taco shells or tortillas, topped with mango salsa. Enjoy!

Serving Size: 1/2 cup
Calories: 320

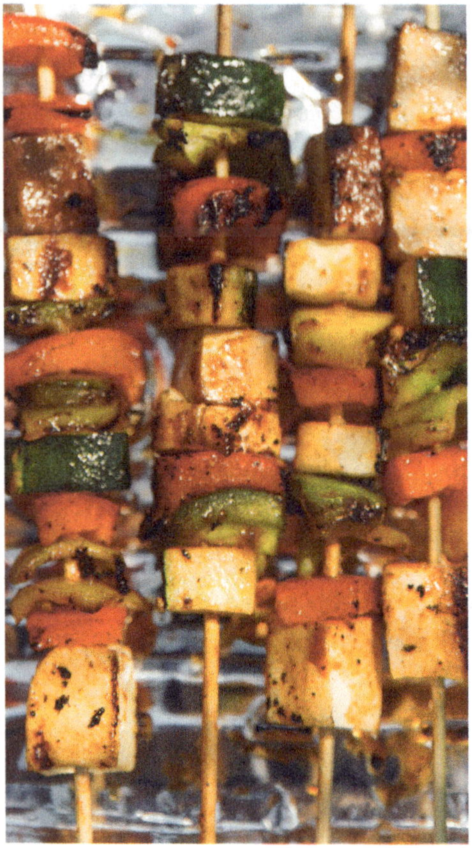

TUNA TERIYAKI KABOBS WITH BROWN RICE

Ingredients:

- 1/2 pound tuna steak, cut into 1-inch cubes
- 1/4 cup low-sodium soy sauce
- 2 cloves garlic, minced
- 1 teaspoon ground ginger
- Salt (optional) and black pepper (optional) to taste

For the kabobs:

- 1 red onion, cut into 1-inch pieces
- 1 green bell pepper, cut into 1-inch pieces
- 1 yellow bell pepper, cut into 1-inch pieces

Instructions:

1. In a large bowl, whisk together soy sauce, garlic, ginger, salt and black pepper (optional). Add tuna cubes and toss to coat. Let marinate for 30 minutes.
2. Preheat grill to medium-high heat.
3. To make kabobs, thread tuna, red onion, green bell pepper, and yellow bell pepper onto skewers. Grill for 5-7 minutes per side, or until tuna is cooked through and vegetables are slightly charred.
4. Serve with brown rice and enjoy!

Serving Size: 1/2 cup
Calories: 330

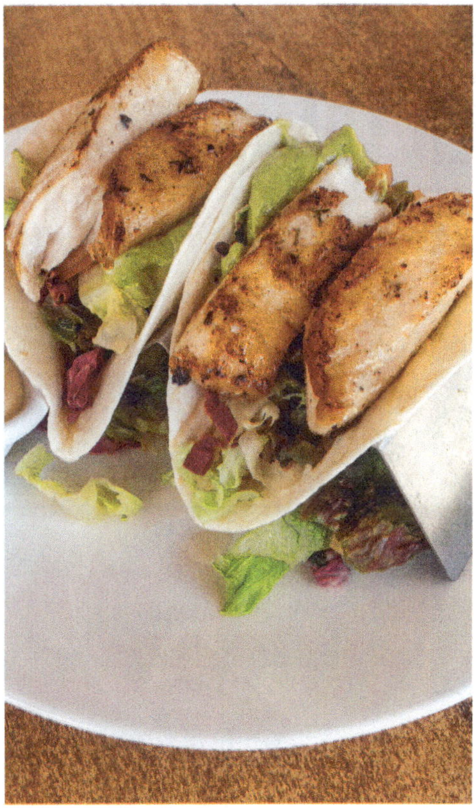

FISH TACOS WITH BERRY SALSA

Ingredients:

- 1/2 pound white fish (such as cod, tilapia, or halibut), cut into 1-inch cubes
- 1 tablespoon olive oil
- Salt (optional) and black pepper (optional) to taste

For the berry salsa:

- 1 cup mixed berries (strawberries, raspberries, blueberries, etc.), diced
- 1/4 red onion, diced
- 2 tablespoons chopped fresh cilantro leaves
- 1 tablespoon freshly squeezed lime juice
- Chopped Lettuce (Optional Sub)

Instructions:

1. Heat a large skillet over medium-high heat. Add fish, olive oil, salt and black pepper (optional) to the skillet. Cook for 5-7 minutes per side, or until fish is cooked through.
2. Meanwhile, in a medium bowl, mix together berries, red onion, cilantro, and lime juice. Season with salt and black pepper (optional) to taste.
3. When fish is cooked through, remove from heat and let cool for 5 minutes. Using two forks, shred the fish.
4. Serve shredded fish on soft taco shells or tortillas, topped with berry salsa. Enjoy!

Serving Size: 1/2 cup
Calories: 350

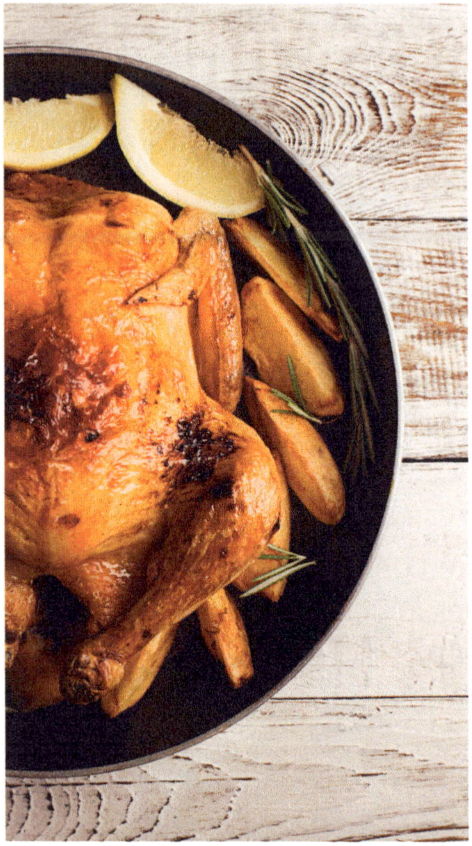

CHICKEN WITH FIRE-ROASTED TOMATOES AND QUINOA

Ingredients:

- 1 tablespoon olive oil
- 1 pound boneless, skinless chicken breast, cut into 1-inch cubes
- Rotisserie chicken (Optional Sub)
- Salt (optional) and black pepper (optional) to taste
- 1/2 teaspoon dried oregano
- 1/2 teaspoon dried thyme
- 1/4 teaspoon paprika
- 1 (14.5 ounce) can diced fire-roasted tomatoes, undrained
- 1 cup quinoa, cooked according to package instructions

Instructions:

1. Heat a large skillet over medium-high heat. Add olive oil, chicken, salt and black pepper (optional), oregano, thyme, and paprika to the skillet. Cook for 6-8 minutes, or until chicken is cooked through.
2. Add fire-roasted tomatoes (undrained) to the skillet. Cook for 2-3 minutes, or until heated through.
3. Serve chicken and sauce over cooked quinoa. Enjoy!

Serving Size: 1 cup
Calories: 350

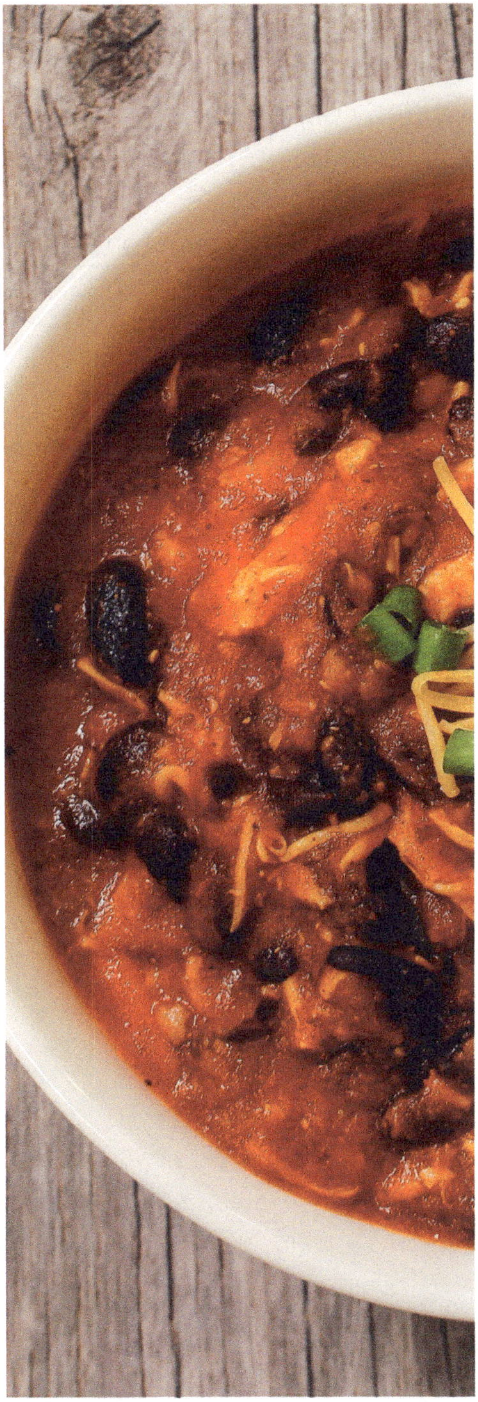

TURKEY CHILI WITH SWEET POTATOES

Ingredients:

- 1 tablespoon olive oil
- 1 pound ground turkey
- 1 onion, diced
- Salt (optional) and black pepper (optional) to taste
- 2 cloves garlic, minced
- 1 teaspoon chili powder
- 1 teaspoon ground cumin
- 1/2 teaspoon dried oregano
- 1/4 teaspoon paprika
- 1/4 teaspoon cayenne pepper (optional)
- 1 (15 ounce) can kidney beans, drained and rinsed
- 1 (14.5 ounce) can diced tomatoes, undrained
- 1 (8 ounce) can tomato sauce

Instructions:

1. Heat a large pot over medium-high heat. Add olive oil, ground turkey, onion, salt and black pepper (optional), garlic, chili powder, cumin, oregano, paprika, and cayenne pepper (optional). Cook for 6-8 minutes, or until turkey is cooked through.
2. Add kidney beans, diced tomatoes (undrained), and tomato sauce to the pot. Stir until well combined. Bring to a boil.
3. Reduce heat to low and let simmer for 10-15 minutes, or until heated through.
4. Serve with brown rice or tortilla chips and enjoy!

Serving Size: 1 cup
Calories: 400

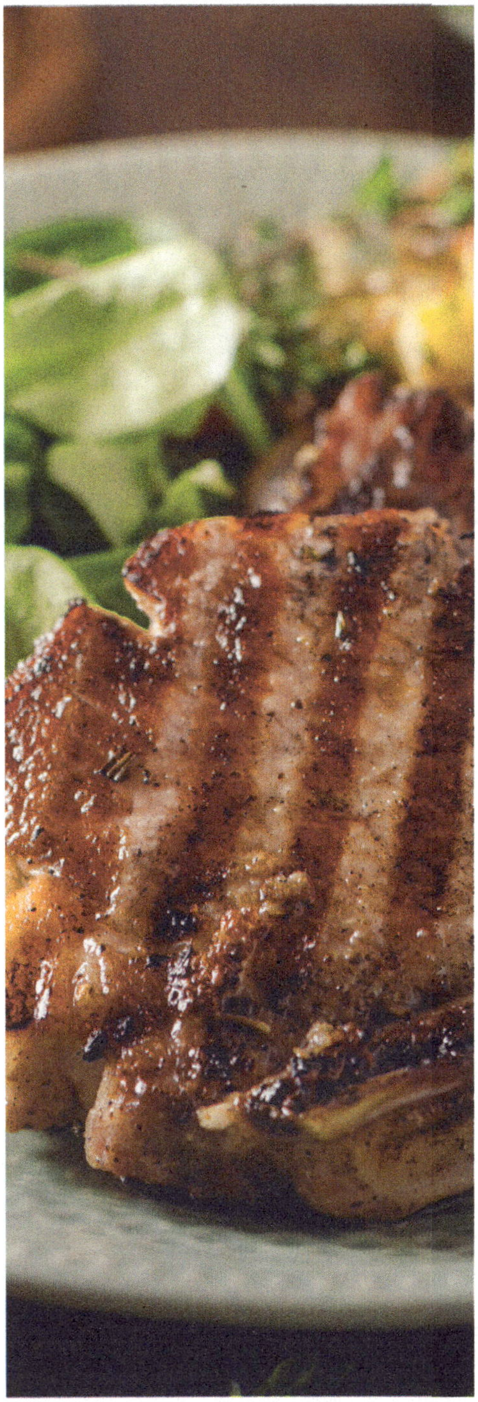

GRILLED PORK NOODLE SALAD

Ingredients:

- 3/4 pound pork tenderloin, trimmed and cut into 1-inch cubes
- 1 tablespoon olive oil
- Salt (optional) and black pepper (optional) to taste
- 2 cloves garlic, minced
- 1/4 teaspoon ground ginger
- 1/8 teaspoon cayenne pepper (optional)
- 3 green onions, thinly sliced
- 6 ounces uncooked whole wheat noodles
- 1 cup snow peas, trimmed

For the dressing:

- 3 tablespoons rice vinegar
- 2 tablespoons freshly squeezed lime juice
- 1 tablespoon sugar-free honey substitute

Instructions:

1. In a large bowl, mix together pork cubes, olive oil, salt and black pepper (optional), garlic, ginger, and cayenne pepper (optional). Let marinate for 15-20 minutes.
2. Preheat grill to medium-high heat.
3. Add pork cubes to grill and cook for 8-10 minutes, or until cooked through. Remove from grill and let cool for 5 minutes.
4. Meanwhile, cook noodles according to package instructions. In the last minute of cooking, add snow peas to the pot. Drain and rinse with cold water.
5. In a small bowl, whisk together rice vinegar, lime juice, honey substitute, salt and black pepper (optional) to taste.
6. In a large serving bowl, combine cooked noodles, snow peas, grilled pork cubes, green onions, and dressing. Toss until well mixed. Serve and enjoy!

Serving Size: 1 cup
Calories: 360

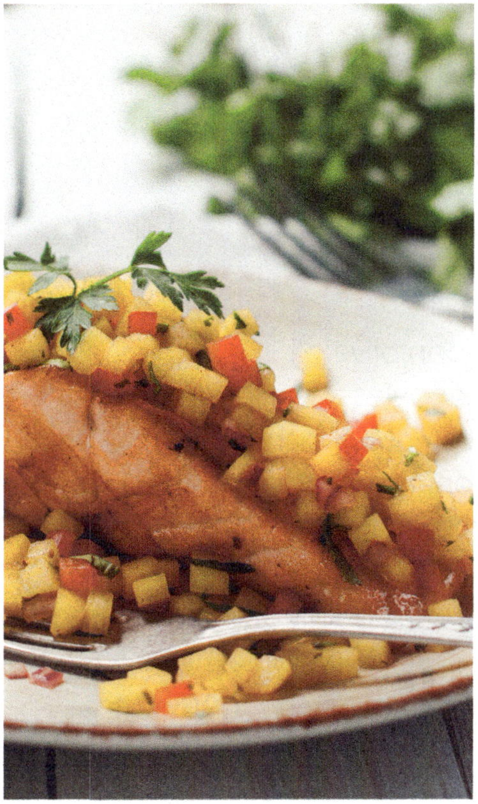

SALMON WITH MANGO SALSA

Ingredients:

- 1 tablespoon olive oil
- 1 pound salmon filets
- Salt (optional) and black pepper (optional) to taste

For the salsa:

- 1 mango, peeled and diced
- 1 avocado, diced
- 1/2 red onion, diced
- 1 jalapeño pepper, seeded and diced
- 3 tablespoons chopped fresh cilantro leaves
- 1 tablespoon freshly squeezed lime juice

Instructions:

1. Preheat grill to medium-high heat.
2. In a small bowl, mix together all of the ingredients for the salsa. Set aside.
3. Rub salmon filets with olive oil and season with salt and black pepper (optional).
4. Grill salmon for 6-8 minutes per side, or until cooked through.
5. Serve salmon with mango salsa and enjoy!

Serving Size: 1 filet
Calories: 400

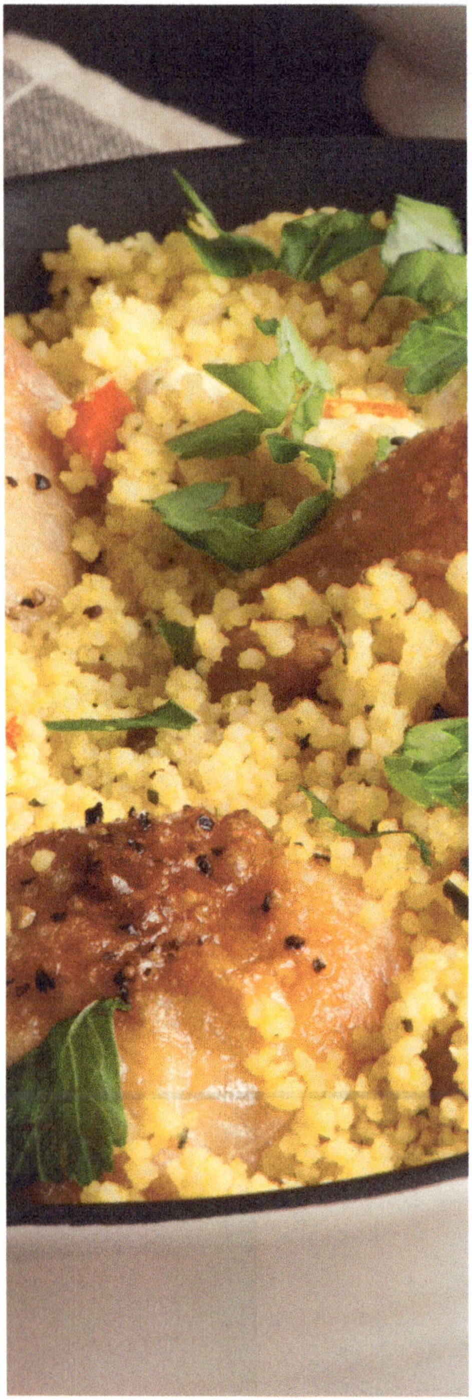

SIMPLE SESAME CHICKEN WITH COUSCOUS

Ingredients:

- 1 tablespoon olive oil
- 1 pound boneless, skinless chicken breasts, cut into 1-inch cubes
- Salt (optional) and black pepper (optional) to taste
- 3 cloves garlic, minced
- 2 tablespoons freshly squeezed lemon juice
- 1 tablespoon sugar-free honey substitute
- 1 tablespoon low-sodium soy sauce
- 1 teaspoon sesame oil
- 1/4 teaspoon crushed red pepper flakes (optional)

Instructions:

1. In a large bowl, whisk together lemon juice, honey substitute, soy sauce, sesame oil, and crushed red pepper flakes (optional).
2. Add chicken cubes to the bowl and coat evenly with the marinade. Let sit for 15-20 minutes.
3. Heat a large skillet over medium-high heat. Add olive oil and chicken cubes to the pan. Cook for 6-8 minutes, or until chicken is cooked through.
4. Serve with couscous and enjoy!

Serving Size: 1 cup
Calories: 400

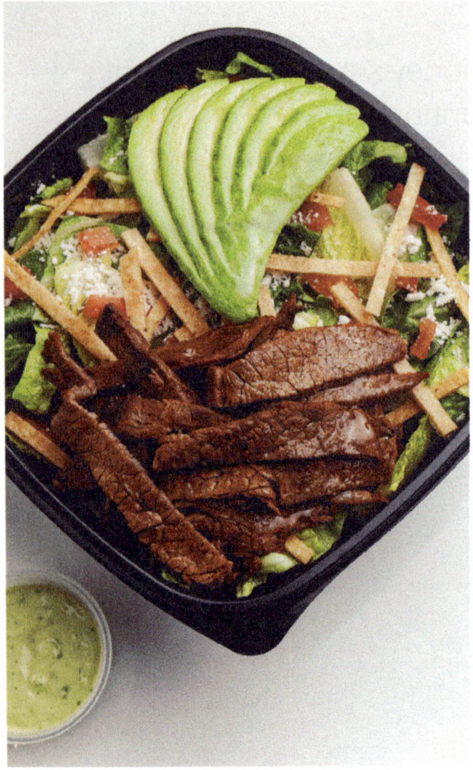

GRILLED STEAK SALAD WITH TOMATOES AND AVOCADO

Ingredients:

- 1 tablespoon olive oil
- 1 pound flank steak, trimmed
- Salt (optional) and black pepper (optional) to taste
- 3 cloves garlic, minced
- 2 tablespoons balsamic vinegar
- 1 tablespoon low-sodium soy sauce
- 2 avocados, diced
- 4 cups mixed salad greens
- 1 pint cherry tomatoes, halved

Instructions:

1. In a large bowl, whisk together balsamic vinegar, soy sauce, and garlic.
2. Rub steak with olive oil and season with salt and black pepper (optional). Add to the bowl and coat evenly with the marinade. Let sit for 15-20 minutes.
3. Preheat grill to medium-high heat.
4. Grill steak for 6-8 minutes per side, or until cooked to desired doneness. Remove from grill and let rest for 5 minutes before slicing into thin strips.
5. In a large serving bowl, combine salad greens, cherry tomatoes, avocado, and grilled steak strips. Toss until well mixed and serve.

Serving Size: 1 salad
Calories: 420

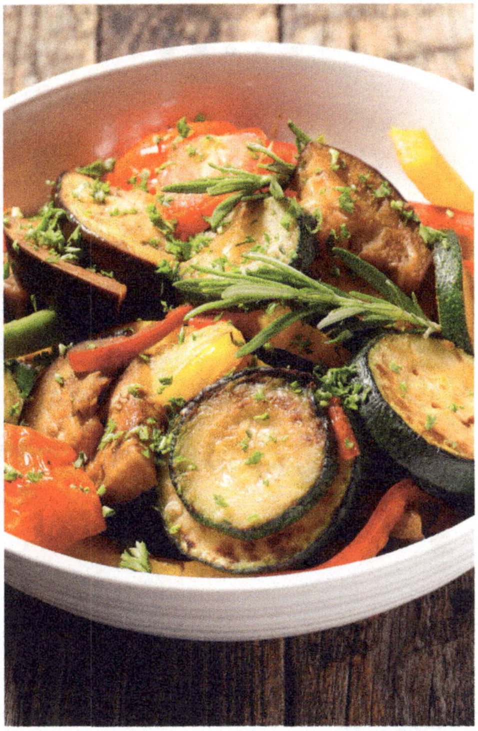

ARTICHOKE RATATOUILLE CHICKEN

Ingredients:

- 1 tablespoon olive oil
- 1 pound boneless, skinless chicken breasts, cut into 1-inch cubes
- Salt (optional) and black pepper (optional) to taste
- 3 cloves garlic, minced
- 2 tablespoons balsamic vinegar
- 1 tablespoon low-sodium soy sauce
- 2 avocados, diced
- 4 cups mixed salad greens
- 1 pint cherry tomatoes, halved

Instructions:

1. In a large bowl, whisk together balsamic vinegar, soy sauce, and garlic.
2. Rub chicken cubes with olive oil and season with salt and black pepper (optional). Add to the bowl and coat evenly with the marinade. Let sit for 15-20 minutes.
3. Preheat grill to medium-high heat.
4. Grill chicken for 6-8 minutes per side, or until cooked through.
5. In a large serving bowl, combine salad greens, cherry tomatoes, avocado, and grilled chicken strips. Toss until well mixed and serve.

Serving Size: 1 salad
Calories: 250

CHAPTER FIVE: Dinners

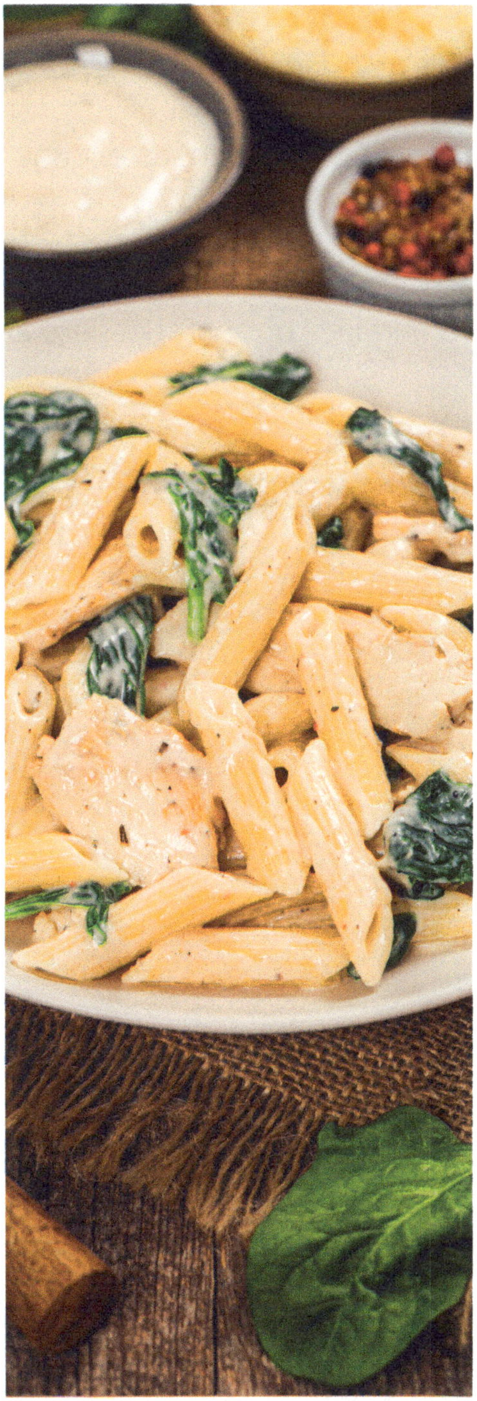

CHICKEN AND SPINACH SKILLET PASTA WITH LEMON AND GARLIC

Ingredients:

- 1 tablespoon olive oil
- 4 cloves garlic, minced
- 1/2 teaspoon crushed red pepper flakes
- 1 pound boneless, skinless chicken breasts, cut into bite-sized pieces
- Salt (optional) and black pepper (optional) to taste
- 3 cups baby spinach leaves
- 1/4 cup chicken broth
- Zest of 1 lemon juice of 1/2 lemon
- 8 ounces whole wheat pasta shells
- 1/4 cup freshly grated Parmesan cheese

Instructions:

1. In a large skillet over medium heat, heat olive oil. Add garlic and red pepper flakes and cook until fragrant.
2. Add chicken and season with salt and black pepper (optional) to taste. Cook until chicken is cooked through and golden brown.
3. Stir in spinach, chicken broth, lemon zest, and lemon juice. Bring to a simmer and cook for 2 minutes, or until spinach is wilted.
4. Add pasta shells and cook for an additional 3-5 minutes, or until shells are al dente.
5. Stir in Parmesan cheese and serve immediately!

Serving Size: 1 bowl
Calories: 610

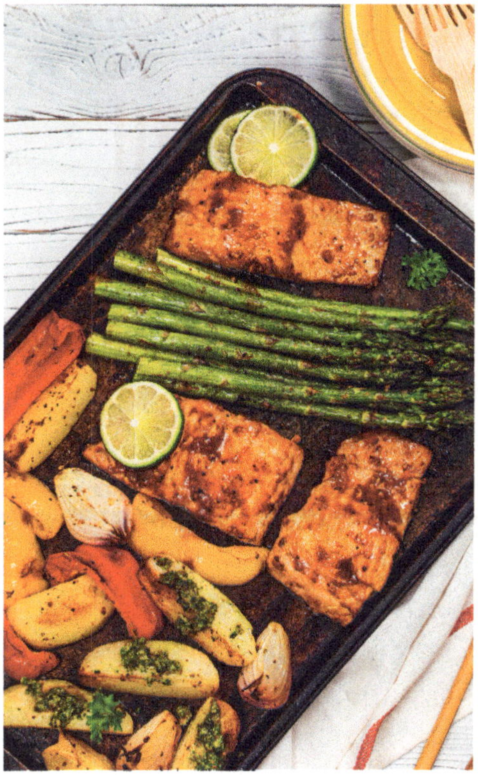

ROASTED SALMON WITH ASPARAGUS AND POTATOES

Ingredients:

- 1 pound fresh asparagus spears, trimmed
- 1 pound Yukon Gold potatoes, cut into bite-sized pieces
- 1/4 cup olive oil
- 4 cloves garlic, minced
- 1 teaspoon dried thyme
- Salt (optional) and black pepper (optional) to taste
- 2 pounds wild-caught salmon filets

Instructions:

1. Preheat oven to 400 degrees F.
2. In a large roasting pan, toss together asparagus, potatoes, olive oil, garlic, thyme, salt and black pepper (optional) to taste.
3. Place salmon filets on top of vegetables and roast for 20-25 minutes, or until salmon is cooked through and vegetables are tender.
4. Serve immediately!

Serving Size: 1 filet with vegetables
Calories: 740

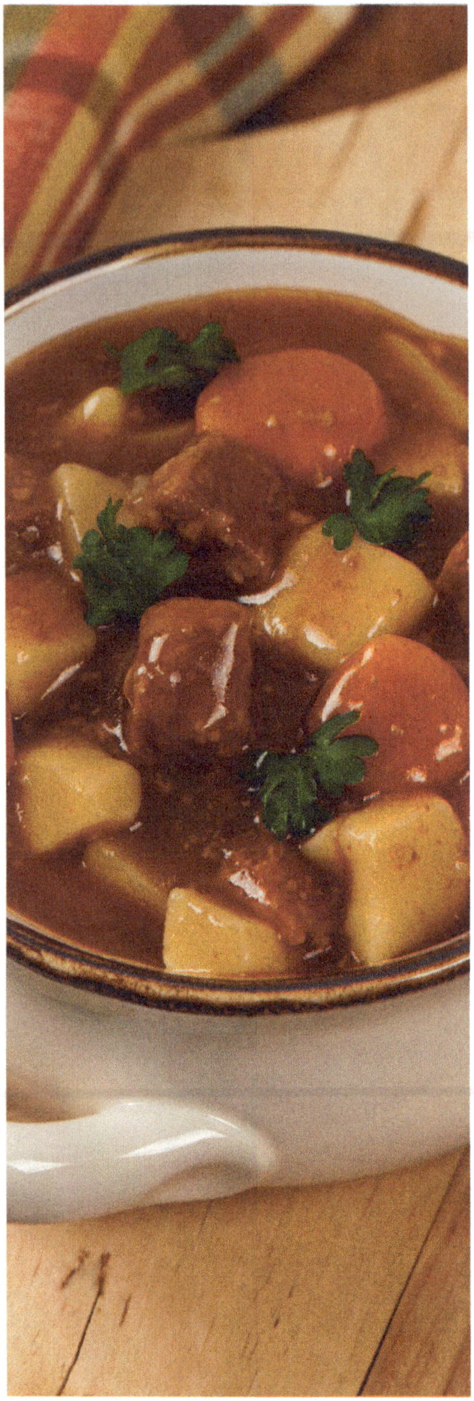

SLOW-COOKER BRAISED BEEF WITH CARROTS AND TURNIPS

Ingredients:

- 3 pounds boneless beef chuck roast, trimmed and cut into bite-sized pieces
- Salt (optional) and black pepper (optional) to taste
- 2 tablespoons olive oil
- 2 cups diced onion
- 6 cloves garlic, minced
- 3 cups low-sodium beef broth
- 1 bay leaf
- 1 tablespoon dried thyme
- 4 large carrots, peeled and cut into 2-inch pieces
- 2 large turnips, peeled and cut into 2-inch pieces

Instructions:

1. Season beef with salt and black pepper (optional) to taste. Heat olive oil in a large Dutch oven over medium heat. Add beef and cook until evenly browned.
2. Stir in onion and garlic and cook for 2 minutes, or until fragrant. Stir in beef broth, bay leaf, and thyme. Bring to a simmer and cook for 3 minutes.
3. Add carrots and turnips and continue cooking until the beef is very tender and the vegetables are cooked through, about 4-6 hours on low or 2-3 hours on high.
4. Remove bay leaf before serving.

Serving Size: 1 cup
Calories: 440

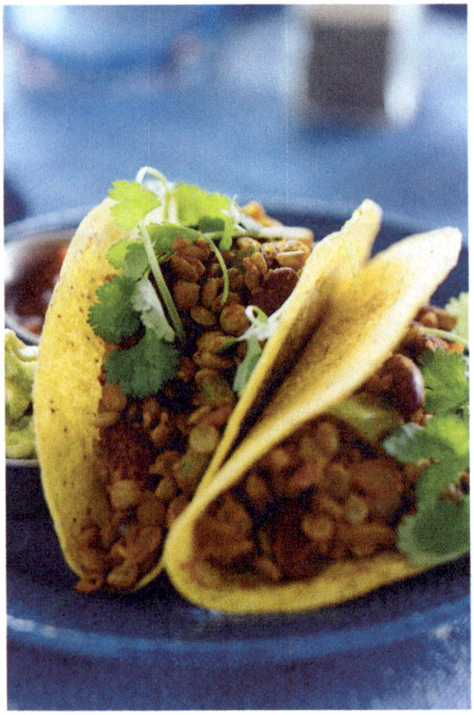

VEGETARIAN LENTIL TACOS

Ingredients:

- 1 tablespoon olive oil
- 1 cup diced onion
- 3 cloves garlic, minced
- 1 cup uncooked green lentils, rinsed and drained
- 1 teaspoon chili powder
- 1 teaspoon ground cumin
- Salt (optional) and black pepper (optional) to taste
- 2 cups water
- 10-12 whole wheat tortillas

Instructions:

1. Heat olive oil in a large saucepan over medium heat. Add onion and garlic and cook until softened, about 5 minutes.
2. Stir in lentils, chili powder, cumin, salt and black pepper (optional) to taste. Pour in water and bring to a boil. Reduce heat to low and simmer for 20-25 minutes, or until lentils are tender.
3. To assemble tacos, place 1/2 cup cooked lentils in the center of each tortilla. Top with shredded lettuce, diced tomatoes, diced onions, and avocado slices (optional).
4. Serve immediately!

Serving Size: 2 tacos
Calories: 210

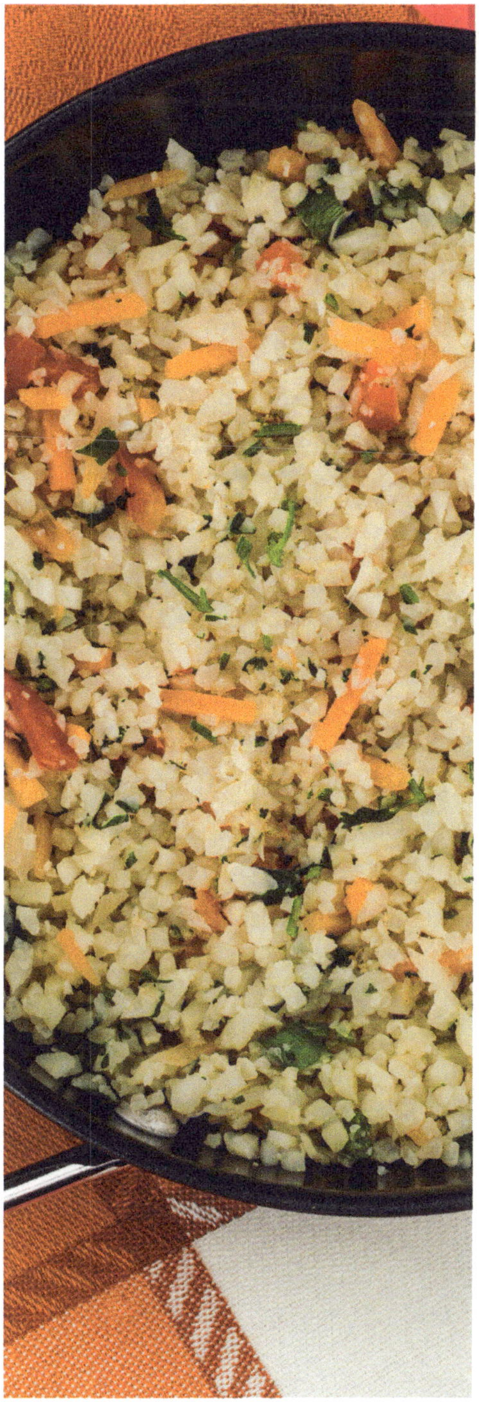

TROPICAL CHICKEN CAULIFLOWER RICE BOWLS

Ingredients:

- 1 tablespoon olive oil
- 1 pound boneless, skinless chicken breasts, cut into bite-sized pieces
- Salt (optional) and black pepper (optional) to taste
- 3 cups riced cauliflower
- 1/2 cup pineapple chunks
- 1 red bell pepper, diced
- 1/4 cup chopped fresh cilantro

Instructions:

1. Heat olive oil in a large skillet over medium heat. Add chicken and season with salt and black pepper (optional) to taste. Cook until chicken is cooked through and golden brown.
2. Stir in riced cauliflower, pineapple chunks, red bell pepper, and cilantro. Cook for 3-5 minutes, or until vegetables are tender.
3. Serve immediately!

Serving Size: 1 bowl
Calories: 400

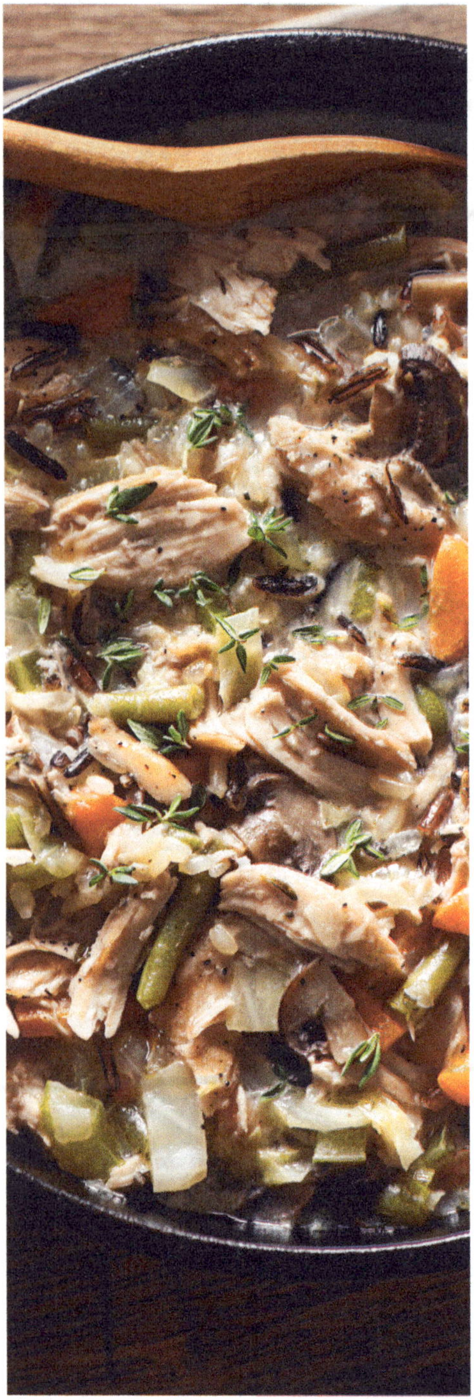

CREAM OF TURKEY AND WILD RICE SOUP

Ingredients:

- 1 tablespoon olive oil
- 1 cup diced onion
- 2 cloves garlic, minced
- 4 cups low-sodium chicken broth
- 1 cup uncooked wild rice, rinsed and drained
- 1 pound cooked turkey, shredded
- 1 cup frozen corn
- Salt (optional) and black pepper (optional) to taste

Instructions:

1. Heat olive oil in a large pot over medium heat. Add onion and garlic and cook until softened, about 5 minutes.
2. Stir in chicken broth and wild rice. Bring to a simmer and cook for 30 minutes, or until the rice is tender.
3. Stir in turkey, corn, salt and black pepper (optional) to taste. Cook for 5 minutes, or until heated through.
4. Serve immediately!

Serving Size: 1 cup
Calories: 330

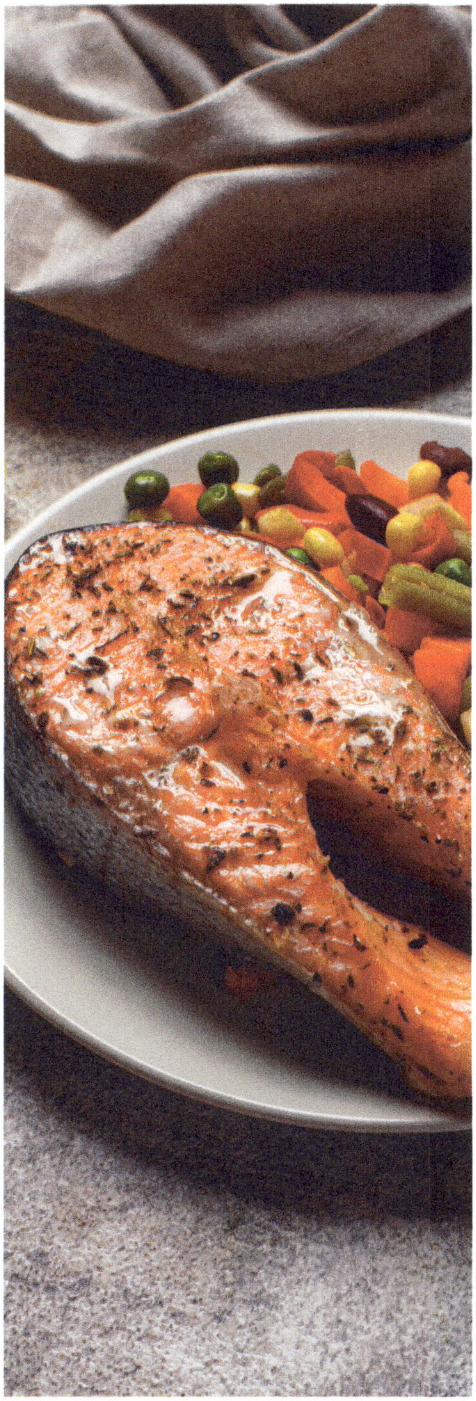

GINGER-TAHINI OVEN-BAKED SALMON AND VEGETABLES

Ingredients:

- 1 pound salmon filets
- Salt (optional) and black pepper (optional) to taste
- 1 tablespoon olive oil
- 1 cup diced onion
- 3 cloves garlic, minced
- 2 cups broccoli florets
- 1 large carrot, peeled and cut into 2-inch pieces
- 1 cup snow peas

For the sauce:

- 3 tablespoons tahini paste
- 2 tablespoons low-sodium soy sauce or tamari
- 1 tablespoon rice vinegar
- 1 tablespoon honey
- 1 teaspoon freshly grated ginger

Instructions:

1. Preheat oven to 400 degrees F.
2. Season salmon filets with salt and black pepper (optional) to taste. Heat olive oil in a large oven-proof skillet over medium heat. Add salmon and cook for 2-3 minutes per side, or until golden brown.
3. Remove salmon from the skillet and set aside. In the same skillet, add onion and garlic and cook until softened, about 5 minutes.
4. Stir in broccoli, carrot, snow peas, and salt (optional) to taste. Cook for 3-5 minutes, or until vegetables are slightly tender.
5. Meanwhile, whisk together tahini paste, soy sauce or tamari, rice vinegar, honey, and ginger in a small bowl until well combined.
6. Return salmon to the skillet and spoon the sauce over top. Bake for 10-12 minutes, or until the salmon is cooked through.
7. Serve immediately!

Serving Size: 1 filet
Calories: 400

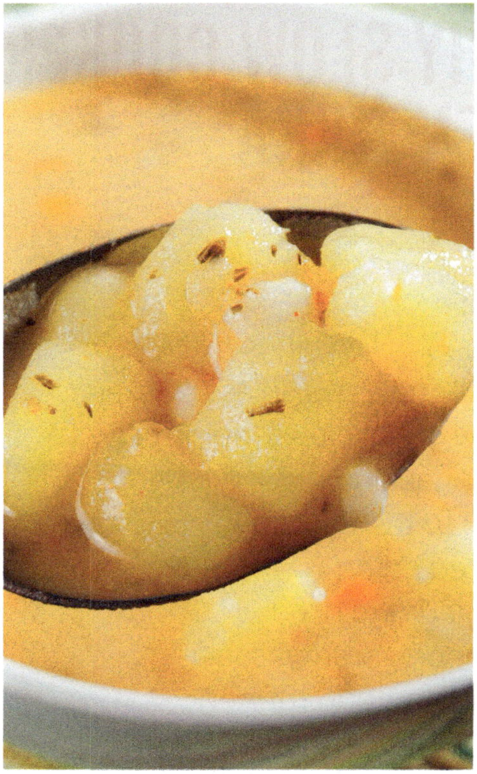

SPICY SAUSAGE AND POTATO SOUP

Ingredients:

- 1 tablespoon olive oil
- 1 pound hot Italian sausage, casing removed
- 1 cup diced onion
- 3 cloves garlic, minced
- 4 cups low-sodium chicken broth
- 2 large russet potatoes, peeled and diced
- 1/2 teaspoon crushed red pepper flakes (optional)
- Salt (optional) and black pepper (optional) to taste

Instructions:

1. Heat olive oil in a large pot over medium heat. Add sausage and cook until browned, about 5 minutes.
2. Stir in onion and garlic and cook until softened, about 5 minutes.
3. Stir in chicken broth, potatoes, crushed red pepper flakes (optional), salt and black pepper (optional) to taste. Bring to a simmer and cook for 15-20 minutes, or until the potatoes are tender.
4. Serve immediately!

Serving Size: 1 cup
Calories: 375

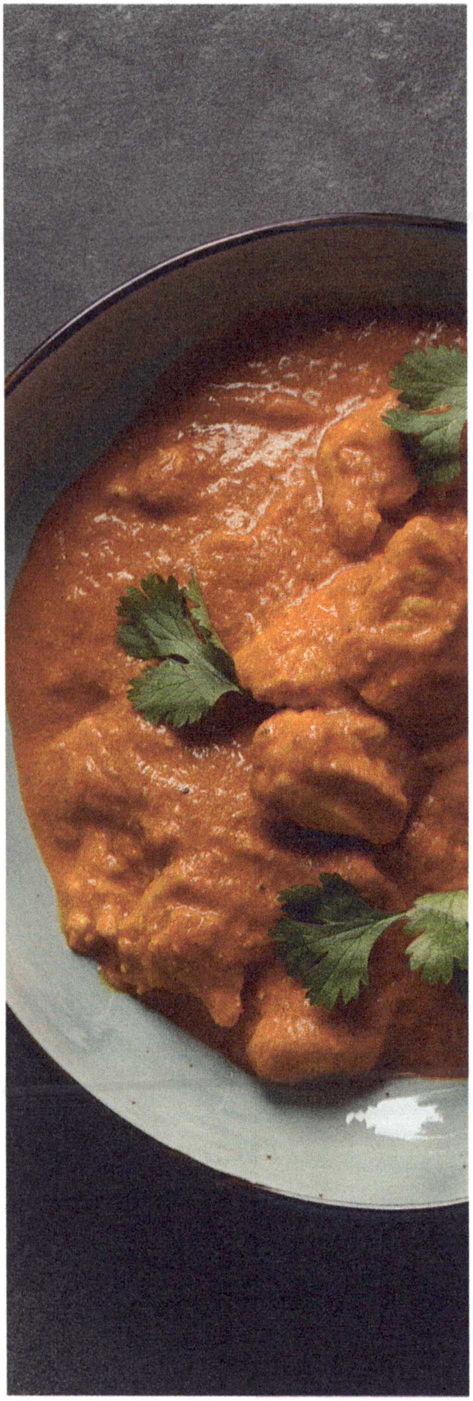

HEALTHY SLOW COOKER CHICKEN TIKKA MASALA

Ingredients:

- 1 tablespoon olive oil
- 1 pound boneless, skinless chicken breasts, cut into bite-sized pieces
- Salt (optional) and black pepper (optional) to taste
- 1 cup diced onion
- 2 cloves garlic, minced
- 1 tablespoon garam masala
- 1 teaspoon ground turmeric
- 1 teaspoon ground cumin
- 1/2 teaspoon ground cinnamon
- 1 (15-ounce) can tomato sauce
- 1 cup plain yogurt

Instructions:

1. Heat olive oil in a large skillet over medium heat. Add chicken and season with salt and black pepper (optional) to taste. Cook until browned, about 5 minutes.
2. Stir in onion and garlic and cook until softened, about 5 minutes.
3. Stir in garam masala, turmeric, cumin, and cinnamon and cook for 1 minute until fragrant.
4. Stir in tomato sauce and yogurt. Bring to a simmer and cook for 5 minutes, or until heated through.
5. Transfer the mixture to a slow cooker and cook on low for 4 hours, or until the chicken is cooked through.
6. Serve immediately!

Serving Size: 1 cup
Calories: 420

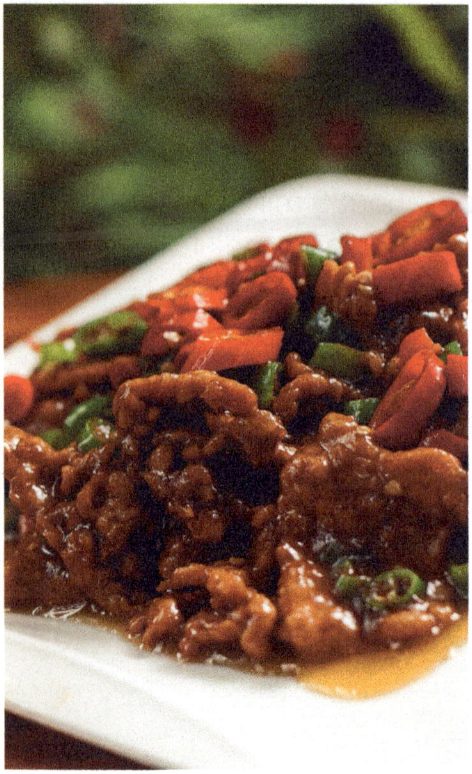

SPICY BEEF & PEPPER STIR-FRY

Ingredients:

- 1 tablespoon olive oil
- 1 pound lean ground beef
- Salt (optional) and black pepper (optional) to taste
- 1 cup diced onion
- 3 cloves garlic, minced
- 1 red bell pepper, diced
- 1 green bell pepper, diced
- 1 jalapeño pepper, seeded and diced
- 2 tablespoons low-sodium soy sauce or tamari
- 2 tablespoons rice vinegar

Instructions:

1. Heat olive oil in a large skillet over medium heat. Add ground beef and season with salt and black pepper (optional) to taste. Cook until browned, about 5 minutes.
2. Stir in onion and garlic and cook until softened, about 5 minutes.
3. Add bell peppers and jalapeño pepper and cook for 3-5 minutes, or until slightly tender.
4. Stir in soy sauce or tamari and rice vinegar. Cook for 1 minute, or until heated through.
5. Serve immediately!

Serving Size: 1 cup
Calories: 350

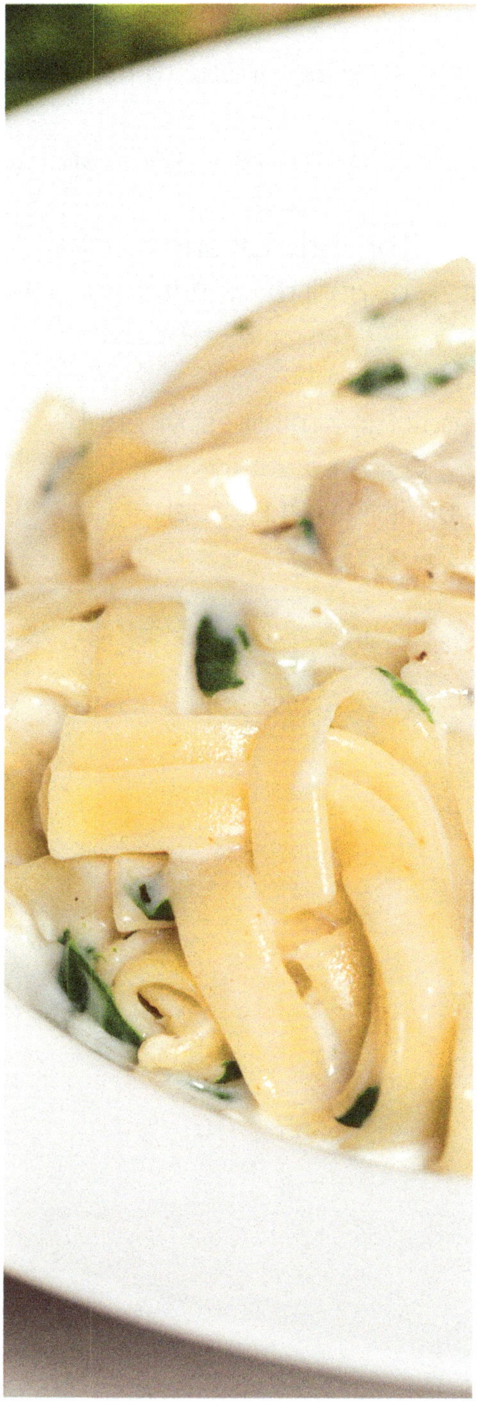

CREAMY FETTUCCINE WITH BRUSSELS SPROUTS AND MUSHROOMS

Ingredients:

- 8 ounces whole wheat fettuccine noodles
- 1 tablespoon olive oil
- 1 cup diced onion
- 3 cloves garlic, minced
- 8 ounces mushrooms, sliced
- 2 cups Brussels sprouts, trimmed and halved (optional)
- Salt (optional) and black pepper (optional) to taste
- 1/4 cup whole wheat flour
- 2 cups low-sodium chicken broth
- 1/2 cup heavy cream

Instructions:

1. Cook fettuccine noodles in a large pot of boiling water according to package instructions.
2. Heat olive oil in a large skillet over medium heat. Add onion and garlic and cook until softened, about 5 minutes.
3. Stir in mushrooms and Brussels sprouts and season with salt and black pepper (optional) to taste. Cook for 5-7 minutes, or until the vegetables are tender.
4. Stir in flour and cook for 1 minute until slightly browned.
5. Stir in chicken broth and bring to a simmer. Cook for 2 minutes, or until thickened.
6. Stir in heavy cream and cook for 1 minute, or until heated through.
7. Serve immediately over cooked fettuccine noodles!

Serving Size: 1 cup
Calories: 400

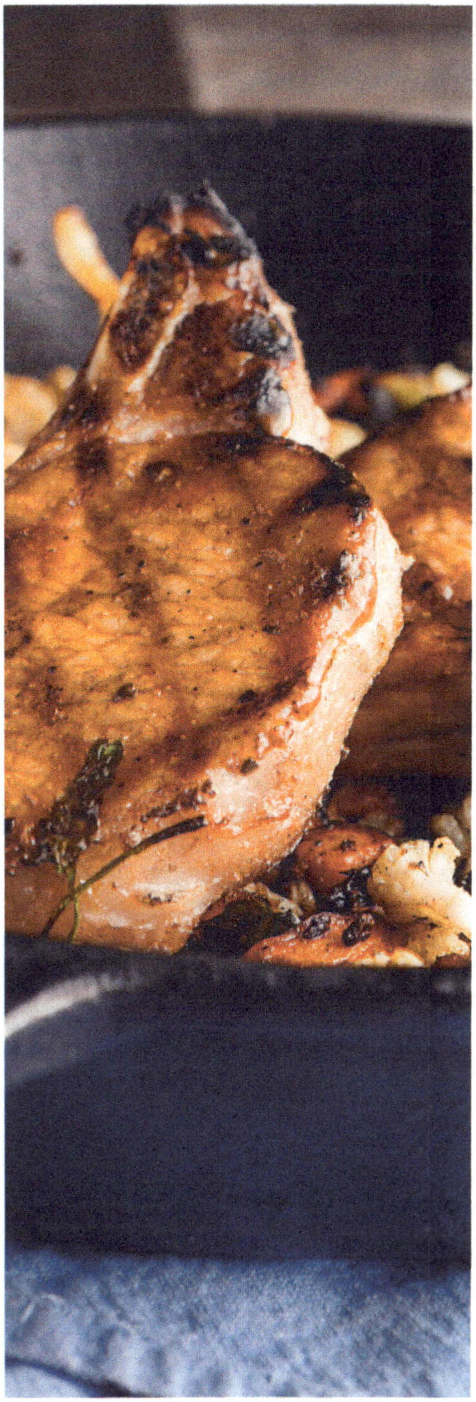

SKILLET PORK CHOPS WITH APPLES AND ONION

Ingredients:

- 4 pork chops
- Salt (optional) and black pepper (optional) to taste
- 1 tablespoon olive oil
- 1 cup diced onion
- 2 cloves garlic, minced
- 2 apples, peeled, cored, and diced

Instructions:

1. Season pork chops with salt and black pepper (optional) to taste.
2. Heat olive oil in a large skillet over medium heat. Add onion and garlic and cook until softened, about 5 minutes.
3. Stir in apples and cook for 3-5 minutes, or until slightly tender.
4. Add pork chops to the skillet and cook for 6-8 minutes per side, or until cooked through.
5. Serve immediately!

Serving Size: 1 pork chop
Calories: 350

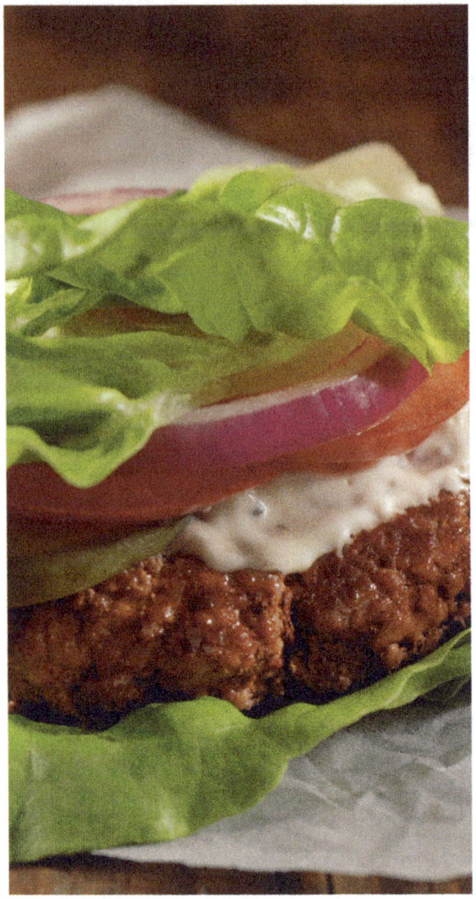

BANH MI CHICKEN BURGER LETTUCE WRAPS

Ingredients:

- 1 pound ground chicken
- Salt (optional) and black pepper (optional) to taste
- 1/4 cup diced onion
- 3 cloves garlic, minced
- 1 carrot, shredded
- 1/4 cup chopped cilantro
- 1 tablespoon low-sodium soy sauce or tamari
- 2 teaspoons sriracha sauce
- 1 teaspoon rice vinegar
- 1/2 teaspoon Stevia
- 8 large lettuce leaves

Instructions:

1. In a large bowl, mix together ground chicken, salt and black pepper (optional), onion, garlic, carrot, cilantro, soy sauce or tamari, sriracha sauce, rice vinegar, and Stevia until well combined.
2. Shape mixture into 8 patties.
3. Heat a grill pan over medium heat and spray with cooking spray.
4. Grill chicken burgers for 5-7 minutes per side, or until cooked through.
5. Serve immediately on lettuce leaves!

Serving Size: 1 chicken burger
Calories: 300

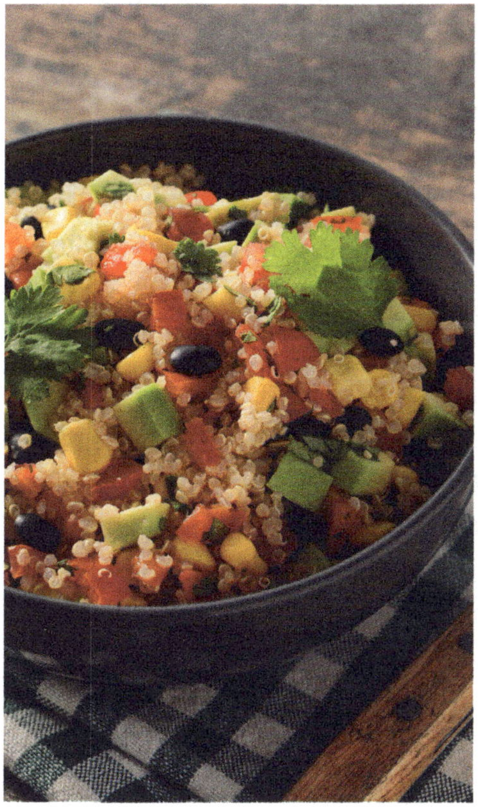

QUINOA BLACK BEAN BURRITO BOWL

Ingredients:

- 1 cup cooked and cooled quinoa
- 1 tablespoon olive oil
- 1 red onion, diced
- 1 red bell pepper, diced
- 1 yellow bell pepper, diced
- 3 cloves garlic, minced
- 1 can (15 ounces) black beans, drained and rinsed
- Salt (optional) and black pepper (optional) to taste
- 1/2 teaspoon chili powder
- 1/2 teaspoon ground cumin
- 1/4 cup chopped fresh cilantro

Instructions:

1. Heat olive oil in a large skillet over medium heat. Add onion and garlic and cook until softened, about 5 minutes.
2. Stir in bell peppers and cook for 3-5 minutes, or until slightly tender.
3. Stir in black beans and season with salt, black pepper (optional), chili powder, and cumin. Cook for 5 minutes, or until heated through.
4. Stir in cooked quinoa and cook for 1-2 minutes, or until heated through.
5. Remove from heat and stir in fresh cilantro. Serve immediately!

Serving Size: 1 cup
Calories: 350

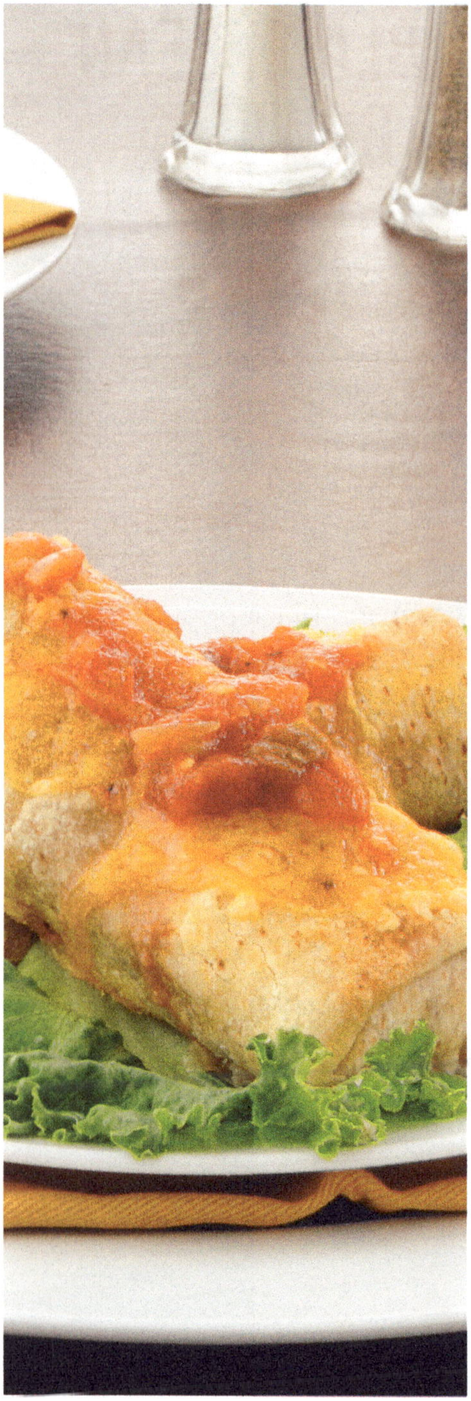

GRILLED BEEF CHIMICHANGAS WITH PICO DE GALLO

Ingredients:

- 1 pound lean ground beef
- Salt (optional) and black pepper (optional) to taste
- 1/2 cup diced onion
- 1/4 cup diced green bell pepper
- 2 cloves garlic, minced
- 1 teaspoon chili powder
- 1 teaspoon ground cumin
- 8 large whole wheat tortillas
- Cooking spray

For the pico de gallo:

- 1 large tomato, diced
- 1/4 cup diced onion
- 1/4 cup chopped fresh cilantro
- Juice of 1 lime

Instructions:

1. Preheat grill to medium-high heat.
2. In a large bowl, mix together ground beef, salt and black pepper (optional), onion, green bell pepper, garlic, chili powder, and cumin.
3. Shape mixture into 8 patties.
4. Grill burgers for 5-7 minutes per side, or until cooked through.
5. Meanwhile, make the pico de gallo: In a medium bowl, mix together diced tomatoes, onion, cilantro, and lime juice.
6. To assemble chimichangas: Lay out each tortilla and place 1 burger in the center. Top with 2 tablespoons of pico de gallo. Fold up the sides of the tortilla and secure with toothpicks if necessary.
7. Spray a large skillet with cooking spray and heat over medium heat. Add chimichangas to the skillet and cook for 2-3 minutes per side, or until lightly browned and crisp.
8. Serve immediately!

Serving Size: 1 chimichanga
Calories: 400

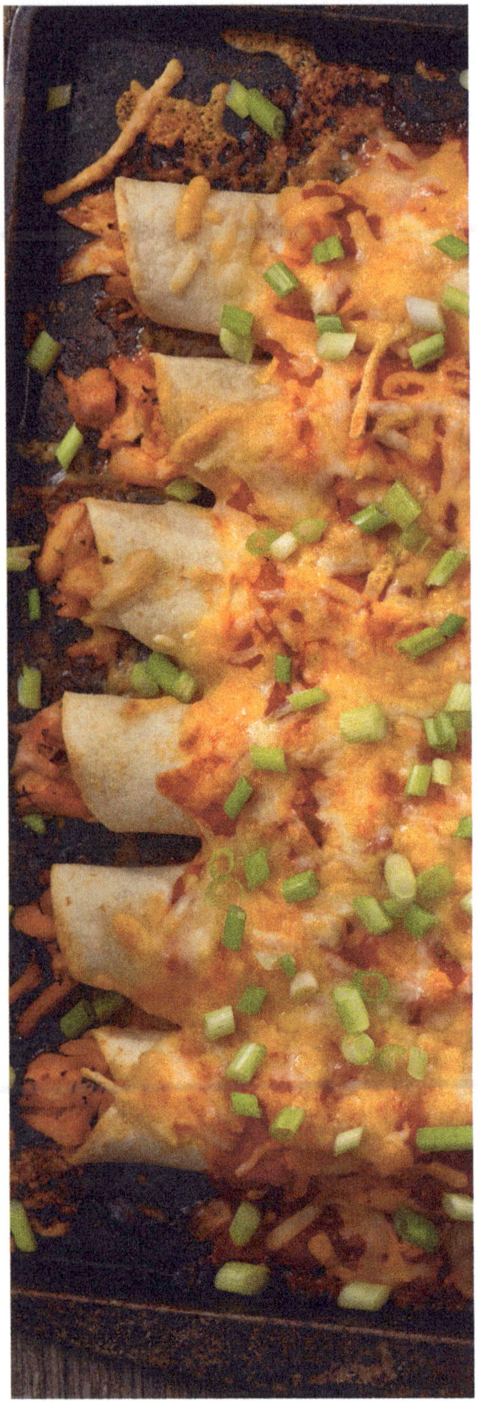

SKINNY CHICKEN ENCHILADAS

Ingredients:

- 1 pound boneless, skinless chicken breasts, cooked and shredded
- Salt (optional) and black pepper (optional) to taste
- 1/2 cup salsa verde
- 1/4 cup diced onion
- 3 cloves garlic, minced
- 1 can (15 ounces) black beans, drained and rinsed
- 1 tablespoon chili powder
- 1 teaspoon ground cumin
- 8 large whole wheat tortillas
- Cooking spray

For the sauce:

- 1/2 cup salsa verde
- 1/2 cup plain nonfat Greek yogurt

Instructions:

1. Preheat oven to 350 degrees F.
2. In a large bowl, mix together chicken, salt and black pepper (optional), salsa verde, onion, garlic, black beans, chili powder, and cumin.
3. Lay out each tortilla and place 1/2 cup of the chicken mixture in the center. Roll up the tortillas and place them seam-side down in a 9x13 inch baking dish that has been sprayed with cooking spray.
4. In a medium bowl, whisk together salsa verde and Greek yogurt. Pour over the top of the enchiladas.
5. Bake for 20-25 minutes, or until heated through.
6. Serve immediately!

Serving Size: 2 enchiladas
Calories: 500

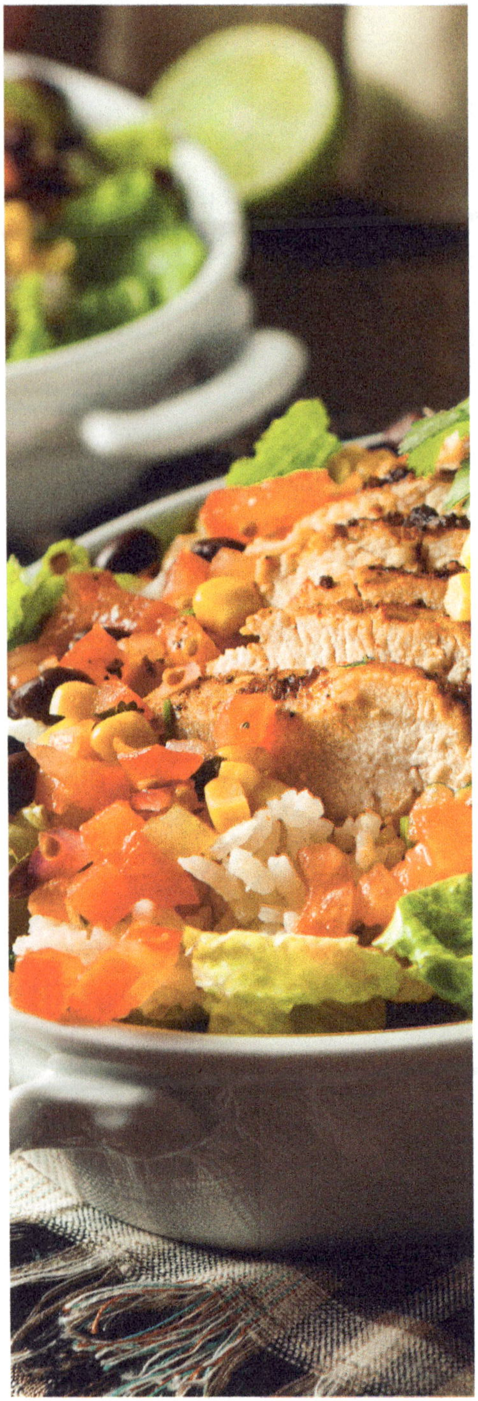

CHICKEN TACO SALAD WITH CILANTRO LIME DRESSING

Ingredients:

- 1 pound boneless, skinless chicken breasts, cooked and shredded
- Salt (optional) and black pepper (optional) to taste
- 1 tablespoon olive oil
- 1/2 cup diced onion
- 1 red bell pepper, diced
- 1 yellow bell pepper, diced
- 3 cloves garlic, minced
- 1 can (15 ounces) black beans, drained and rinsed
- 1/2 teaspoon chili powder
- 1/2 teaspoon ground cumin
- 6 cups chopped Romaine lettuce

For the cilantro lime dressing:

- 1/4 cup plain nonfat Greek yogurt
- 2 tablespoons salsa
- 1 tablespoon olive oil
- 1/4 cup chopped fresh cilantro
- Juice of 1 lime

Instructions:

1. In a large bowl, mix together chicken, salt and black pepper (optional), olive oil, onion, bell peppers, garlic, black beans, chili powder, and cumin.
2. In a small bowl, whisk together Greek yogurt, salsa, olive oil, cilantro, and lime juice.
3. Pour the dressing over the chicken mixture and mix until everything is coated.
4. Serve over a bed of Romaine lettuce and top with fresh cilantro.
5. Enjoy!

Serving Size: 1 salad
Calories: 400

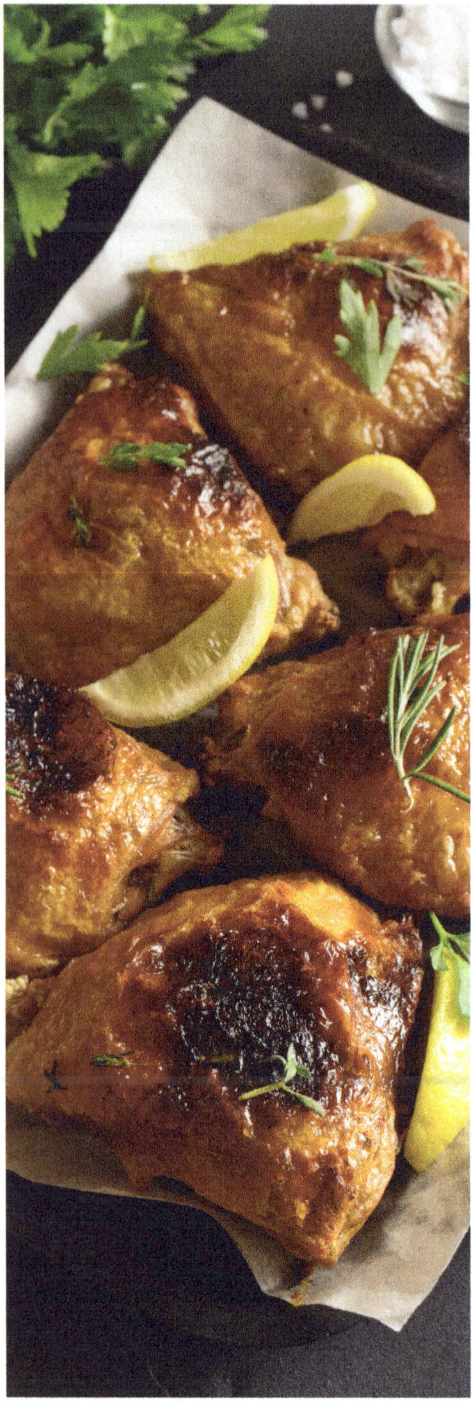

MAPLE-ROASTED CHICKEN THIGHS WITH SWEET POTATO WEDGES AND BRUSSELS SPROUTS

Ingredients:

- 8 chicken thighs
- Salt and black pepper (optional) to taste
- 1 tablespoon olive oil
- 2 cloves garlic, minced
- 1 teaspoon dried thyme
- 3 tablespoons pure maple syrup
- 4 large sweet potatoes, cut into wedges
- Cooking spray
- 1/2 pound Brussels sprouts, trimmed and halved

Instructions:

1. Preheat oven to 425 degrees F.
2. Season chicken thighs with salt and black pepper (optional). In a large bowl, mix together chicken, olive oil, garlic, thyme, and 2 tablespoons of maple syrup. Marinate for at least 30 minutes.
3. Line a baking sheet with foil and place a wire rack on top. Spray the rack with cooking spray. Place chicken on the rack and roast for 25 minutes.
4. While chicken is roasting, place sweet potato wedges on another baking sheet that has been sprayed with cooking spray. Season with salt and black pepper (optional) and roast for 20 minutes.
5. After 20 minutes, add Brussels sprouts to the sweet potatoes and mix everything around so that the Brussels sprouts are coated with a little bit of oil. Roast for an additional 10-15 minutes, or until all vegetables are tender.
6. When chicken is done, brush with remaining maple syrup and let rest for 5 minutes before cutting into it.
7. Serve chicken and vegetables together and enjoy!

Serving Size: 2 chicken thighs with vegetables
Calories: 500

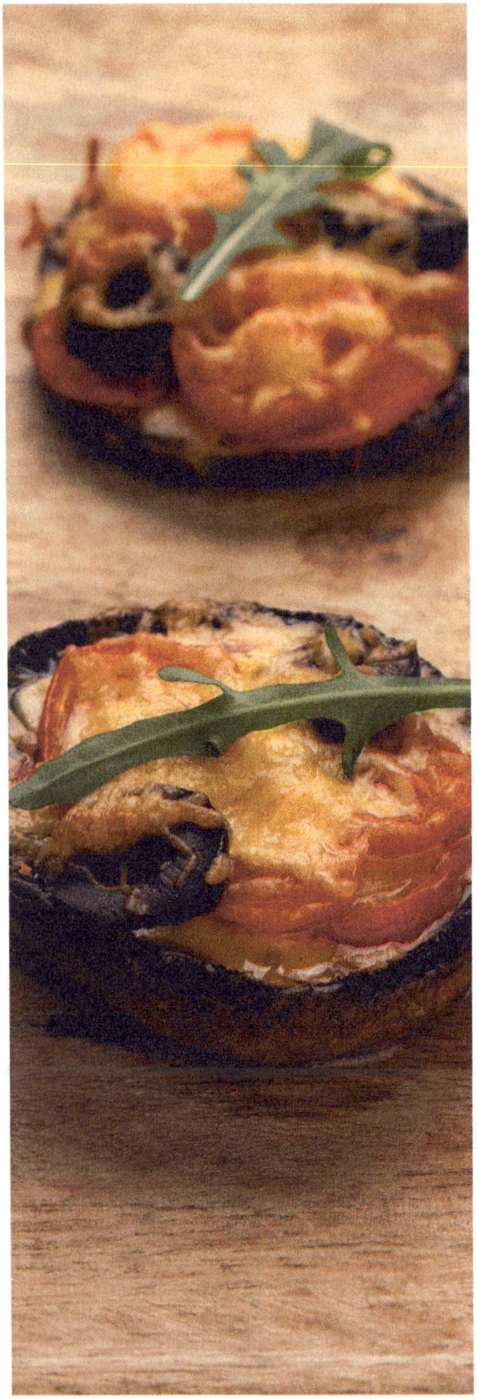

LASAGNA STUFFED PORTOBELLO MUSHROOMS

Ingredients:

- 4 large portobello mushrooms
- 1/2 pound lean ground beef
- 1/2 cup diced onion
- 3 cloves garlic, minced
- Salt and black pepper (optional) to taste
- 1 jar (24 ounces) marinara sauce
- 1 container (15 ounces) part-skim ricotta cheese
- 1 egg, beaten
- 1/4 cup chopped fresh parsley
- 1/2 teaspoon dried oregano
- 1/2 teaspoon dried basil
- 6 lasagna noodles, cooked according to package instructions
- 1 1/2 cups shredded mozzarella cheese

Instructions:

1. Preheat oven to 350 degrees F.
2. In a large skillet over medium heat, cook beef, onion, garlic, salt and black pepper (optional) until beef is browned. Drain any excess fat and remove from heat. Stir in marinara sauce.
3. In a medium bowl, mix together ricotta cheese, egg, parsley, oregano, and basil.
4. Spray a 9×13 inch baking dish with cooking spray.
5. To assemble lasagna: spread 1/2 cup of meat sauce on the bottom of the dish. Top with 3 noodles (break them to fit if necessary), then spread half of the ricotta mixture over the noodles. Sprinkle with 1/2 cup mozzarella cheese. Repeat layering.
6. Cover with foil and bake for 30 minutes. Remove foil and bake for an additional 10-15 minutes, or until lasagna is bubbly and cheese is melted.
7. Let rest for 5-10 minutes before serving. Enjoy!

Serving Size: 1/9th of recipe
Calories: 400

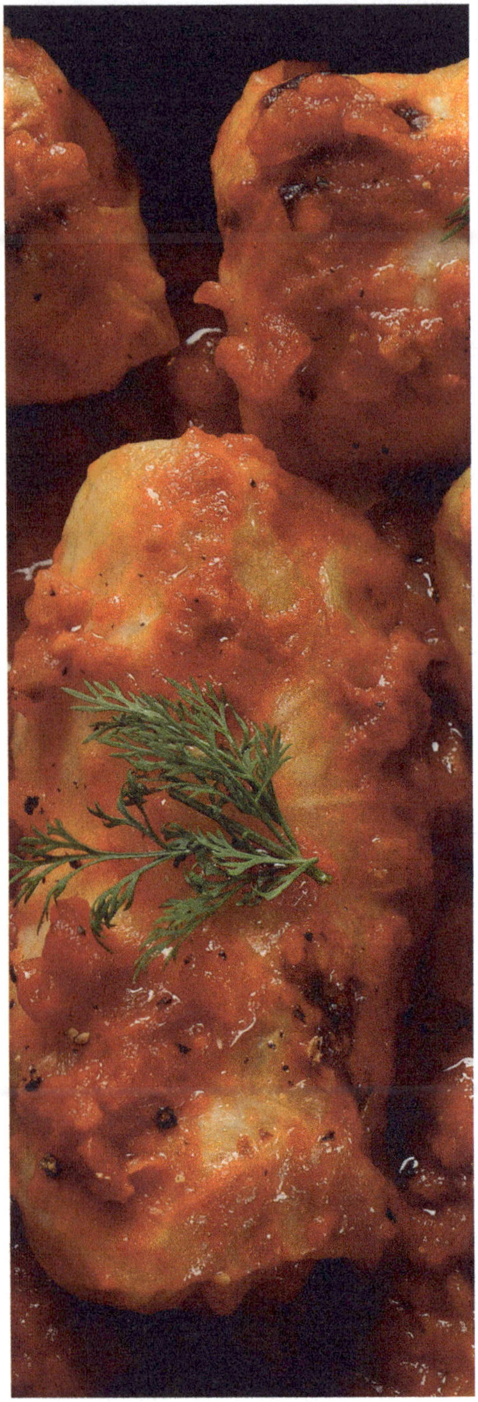

BEEF AND RICE STUFFED CABBAGE ROLLS

Ingredients:

- 1 large head of cabbage
- 1 pound lean ground beef
- 1/2 cup diced onion
- 3 cloves garlic, minced
- Salt and black pepper (optional) to taste
- 1 can (14.5 ounces) diced tomatoes, undrained
- 1 can (8 ounces) tomato sauce
- 1 tablespoon Stevia
- 2 teaspoons dried oregano
- 1 teaspoon smoked paprika
- 1 cup cooked rice

Instructions:

1. Preheat oven to 350 degrees F.
2. In a large pot of boiling water, cook cabbage for 3-4 minutes until leaves are slightly softened. Remove from water and let cool.
3. In a medium bowl, mix together ground beef, onion, garlic, salt and black pepper (optional), diced tomatoes with their juice, tomato sauce, Stevia, oregano, and smoked paprika.
4. To assemble cabbage rolls: take a large cabbage leaf and spoon 1/3 cup of meat mixture in the center. Roll up leaf, tucking in the sides as you go. Place seam side down in a baking dish. Repeat with remaining leaves and meat mixture.
5. Cover dish with foil and bake for 45 minutes. Remove foil and bake for an additional 10-15 minutes, or until cabbage rolls are cooked through.
6. Serve immediately and enjoy!

Serving Size: 2 cabbage rolls
Calories: 440

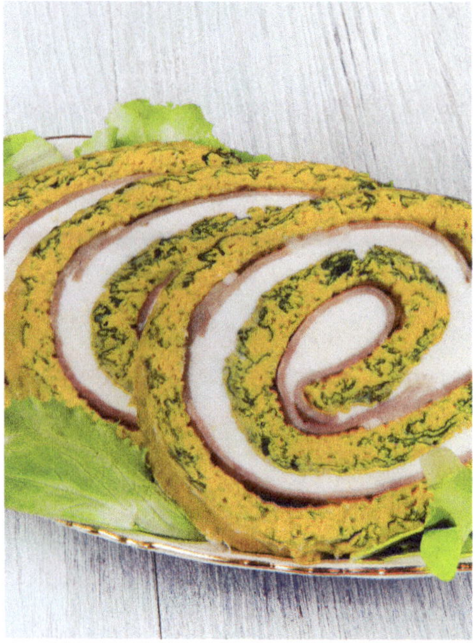

SPINACH ROLLS

Ingredients:

- 1 package (10 ounces) frozen chopped spinach, thawed and squeezed dry
- 1/4 cup diced onion
- 3 cloves garlic, minced
- Salt and black pepper (optional) to taste
- 1 container (15 ounces) part-skim ricotta cheese
- 2 eggs, beaten
- 1/4 cup grated Parmesan cheese
- 1 package (8 ounces) reduced-fat Crescent rolls

Instructions:

1. Preheat oven to 375 degrees F.
2. In a medium bowl, mix together spinach, onion, garlic, salt and black pepper (optional), ricotta cheese, eggs, and Parmesan cheese. Set aside.
3. Separate crescent dough into 8 triangles.
4. To assemble rolls: place a heaping tablespoon of spinach mixture in the center of each triangle. Roll up dough, starting at the wide end, and tucking in the sides as you go. Place seam side down on a baking sheet lined with parchment paper or a silicone baking mat.
5. Bake for 12-15 minutes, or until rolls are golden brown and cooked through. Enjoy!

Serving Size: 2 rolls
Calories: 300

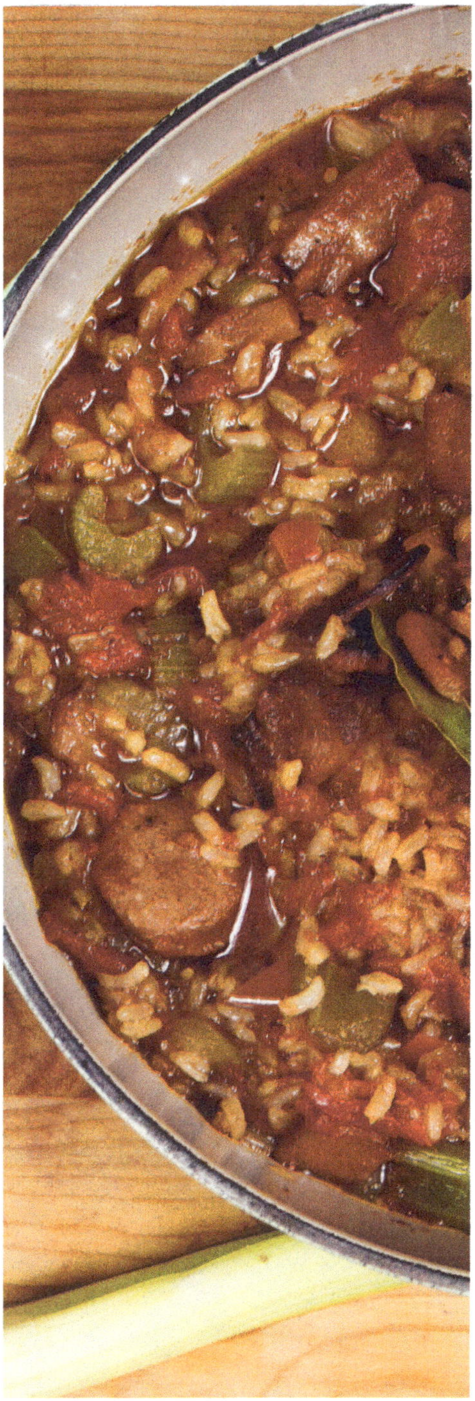

MEATY SLOW-COOKED JAMBALAYA

Ingredients:

- 1 pound lean ground beef
- 1/2 cup diced onion
- 3 cloves garlic, minced
- Salt and black pepper (optional) to taste
- 1 can (14.5 ounces) diced tomatoes, undrained
- 1 can (8 ounces) tomato sauce
- 1 tablespoon Cajun seasoning
- 4 cups cooked rice

Instructions:

1. In a large skillet over medium heat, cook beef, onion, garlic, salt and black pepper until beef is browned. Drain any excess fat and remove from heat. Stir in diced tomatoes with their juice, tomato sauce, Cajun seasoning, and cooked rice.
2. Pour mixture into a slow cooker and stir well. Cover and cook on low for 6-8 hours, or until heated through.
3. Serve immediately and enjoy!

Serving Size: 1 1/2 cups
Calories: 490

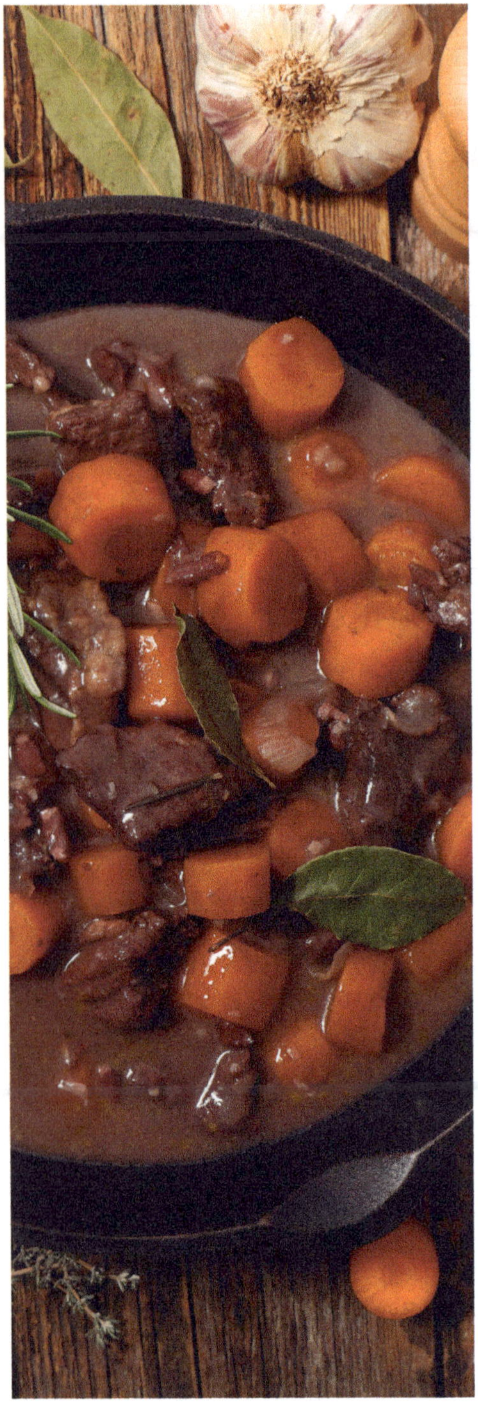

BOEUF BOURGUIGNON

Ingredients:

- 1 1/2 pounds beef stew meat, cut into 1-inch cubes
- Salt and black pepper (optional) to taste
- 3 tablespoons all-purpose flour
- 3 tablespoons olive oil
- 1 large onion, diced
- 4 cloves garlic, minced
- 1 bottle (750 ml) dry red wine
- 2 cups beef broth
- 1 bay leaf
- 2 teaspoons dried thyme leaves
- 8 ounces baby carrots, halved lengthwise
- 16 ounces frozen pearl onions, thawed

Instructions:

1. Preheat oven to 375 degrees F.
2. Season beef with salt and black pepper (optional). Toss with flour to coat.
3. In a large Dutch oven or heavy-duty pot, heat olive oil over medium-high heat. Add beef and cook until browned on all sides. Remove from pot and set aside.
4. To the same pot, add onion and garlic. Cook until softened, stirring occasionally. Pour in red wine and beef broth. Stir in bay leaf and thyme leaves. Return beef to the pot.
5. Cover and bake for 1 1/2 hours, or until beef is almost tender. Stir in baby carrots and pearl onions. Bake for an additional 30 minutes, or until vegetables are tender and stew is thickened.
6. Remove bay leaf before serving. Enjoy!

Serving Size: 1 1/2 cups
Calories: 700

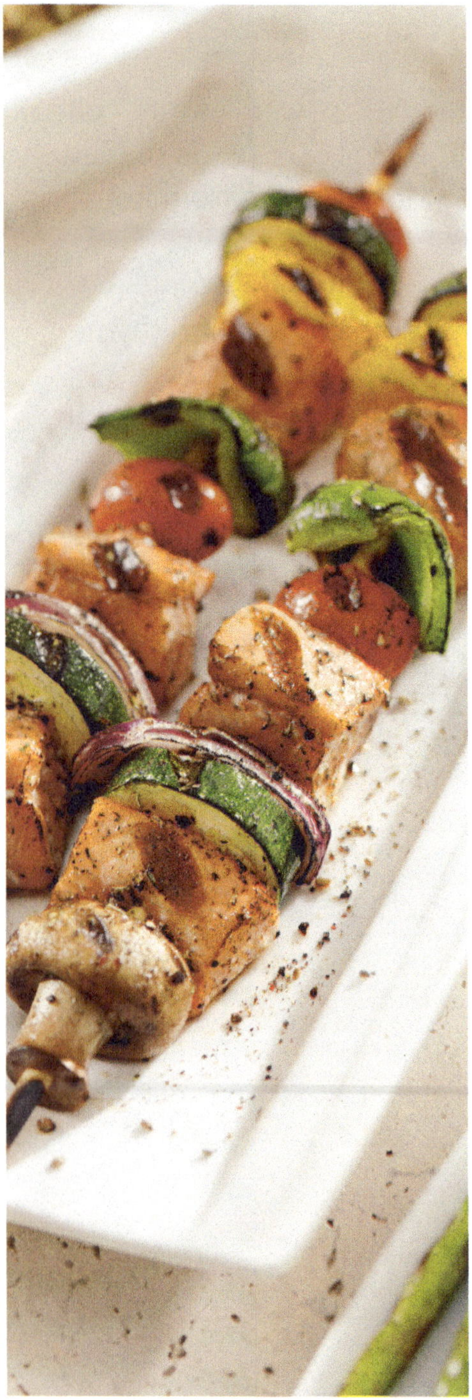

MEDITERRANEAN GRILLED SALMON KABOBS

Ingredients:

- 1 1/2 pounds salmon, cut into 1-inch cubes
- Salt and black pepper (optional) to taste
- 3 tablespoons olive oil, divided
- 2 tablespoons freshly squeezed lemon juice
- 1 tablespoon dried oregano leaves
- 4 cloves garlic, minced
- 1 large red onion, cut into 1-inch pieces
- 1 large green bell pepper, cut into 1-inch pieces
- 1 large yellow bell pepper, cut into 1-inch pieces

Instructions:

1. Preheat grill to medium-high heat.
2. In a large bowl, season salmon with salt and black pepper (optional). Drizzle with 2 tablespoons olive oil and lemon juice. Sprinkle with oregano and garlic, and toss to coat.
3. In a separate bowl, toss together red onion, green bell pepper, and yellow bell pepper with remaining 1 tablespoon olive oil.
4. To assemble kabobs: alternately thread salmon and vegetables onto 8-10 skewers (if using wooden skewers, soak in water for 30 minutes before using).
5. Grill kabobs for 10-12 minutes, or until salmon is cooked through and vegetables are slightly charred. Serve immediately and enjoy!

Serving Size: 2 kabobs
Calories: 600

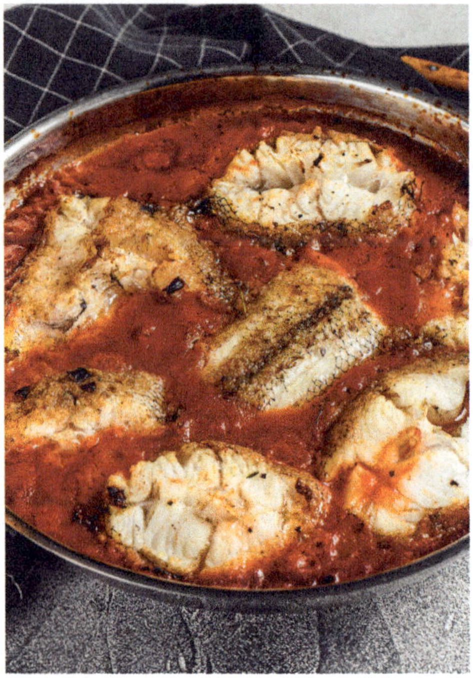

COD WITH HEARTY TOMATO SAUCE

Ingredients:

- 1 tablespoon olive oil
- 4 cloves garlic, minced
- 1 large onion, diced
- Salt and black pepper (optional) to taste
- 2 cans (14.5 ounces each) diced tomatoes, undrained
- 1/4 cup chopped fresh parsley leaves
- 1/4 cup chopped fresh basil leaves
- 4 cod filets (6 ounces each), rinsed and patted dry

Instructions:

1. Preheat oven to 400 degrees F.
2. In a large saucepan or Dutch oven over medium heat, heat olive oil until hot. Add garlic and onion and season with salt and black pepper (optional). Cook until softened, stirring occasionally. Stir in diced tomatoes with their juice, parsley, and basil. Bring to a simmer and cook for 5 minutes.
3. Place cod filets in a single layer in the sauce. Cover and bake for 10-12 minutes, or until fish is cooked through.
4. Serve immediately with crusty bread or over cooked rice or pasta, if desired. Enjoy!

Serving Size: 1 cod filet with 1/2 cup sauce
Calories: 400

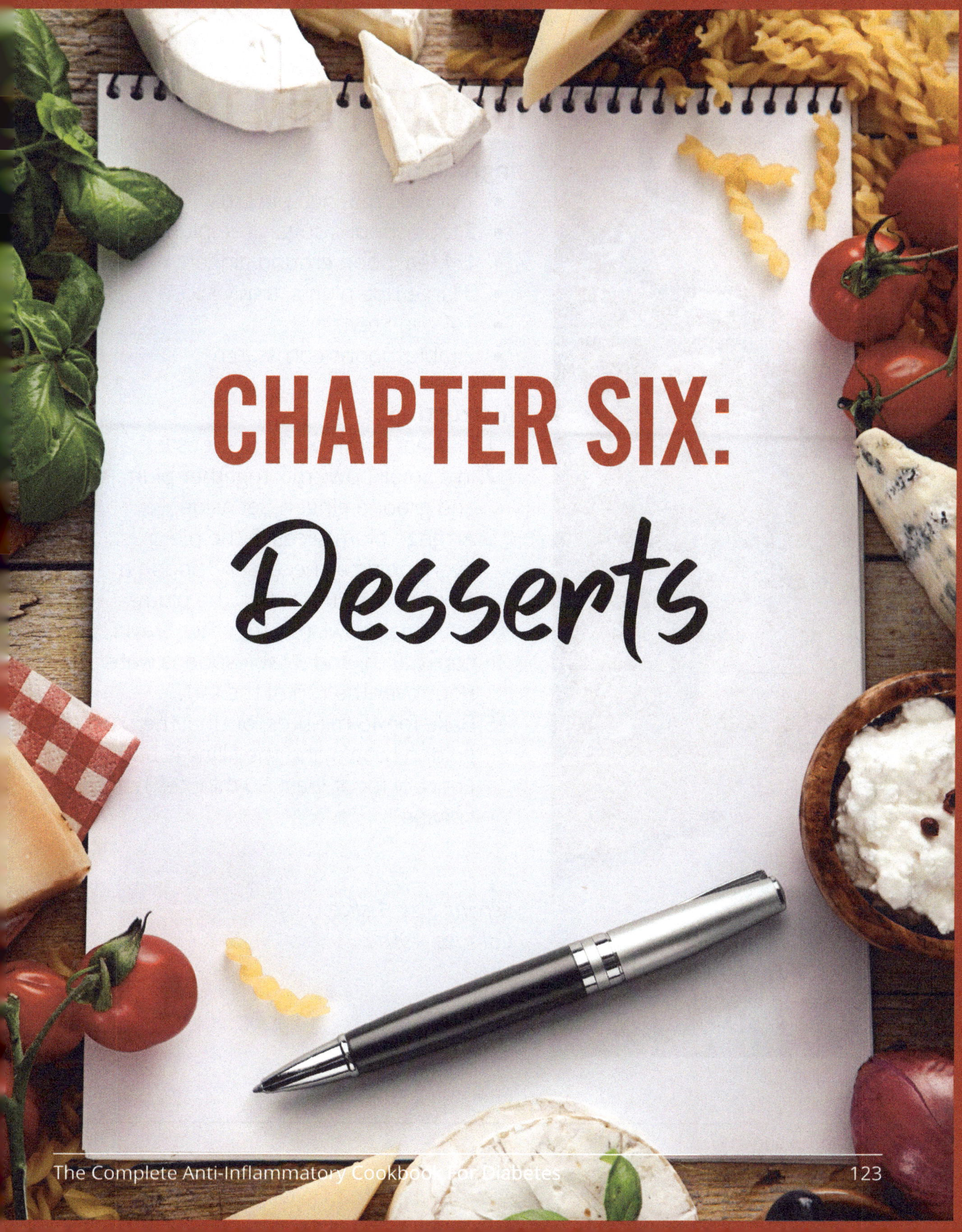

CHAPTER SIX: Desserts

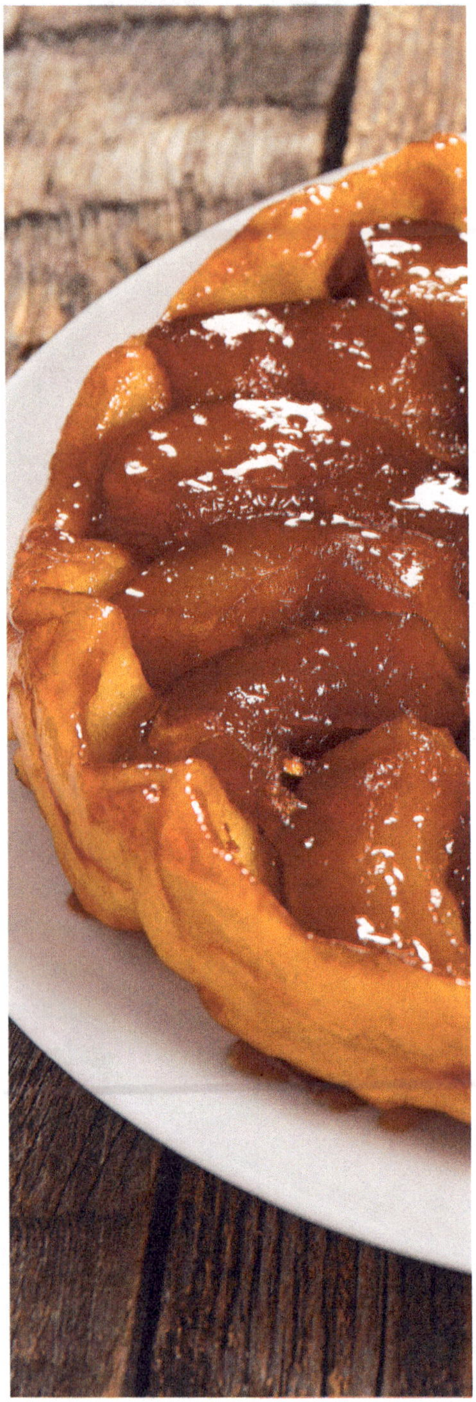

GINGER PLUM TART

Ingredients:

- 1 unbaked 9-inch pie crust
- 2 tablespoons sugar-free plum jam
- 1/4 teaspoon ground ginger
- 3 large ripe plums, thinly sliced
- 1/4 cup Stevia
- 2 tablespoons cornstarch

Instructions:

1. Preheat oven to 375 degrees F.
2. In a small bowl, mix together plum jam and ground ginger. Set aside.
3. Arrange plum slices in the pie crust, overlapping as necessary. Spoon the jam mixture over the top of the plums.
4. In a small bowl, mix together Stevia, cornstarch, and 3 tablespoons water. Pour over the top of the tart.
5. Bake for 45 minutes, or until the crust is golden brown and the filling is bubbly. Let cool for at least 30 minutes before serving.

Serving Size: 1 slice
Calories: 190

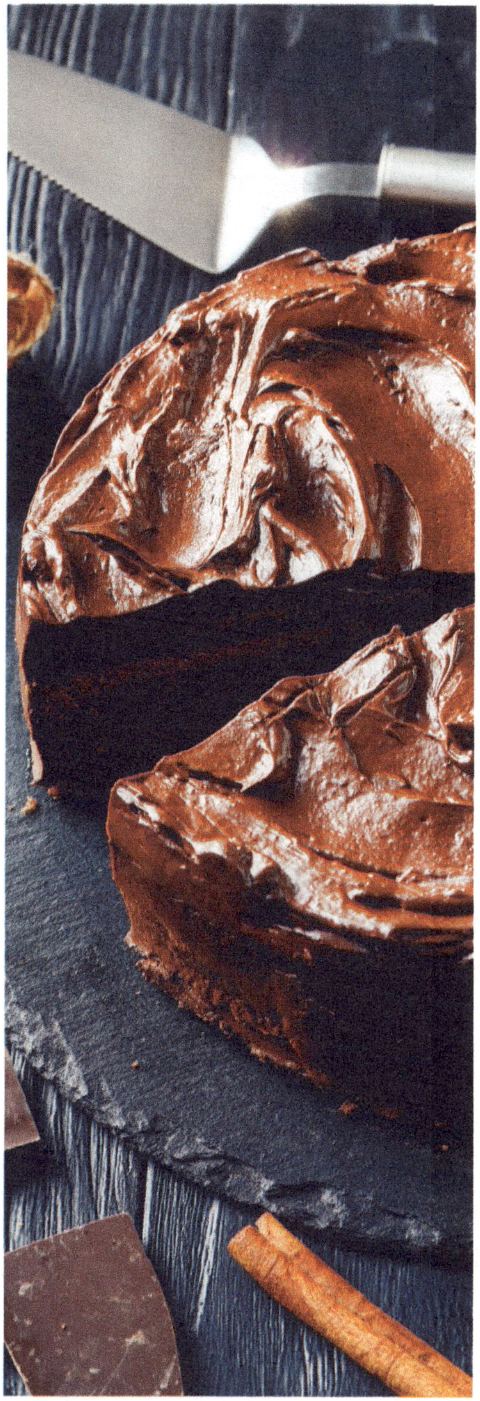

CHOCOLATE CAKE

Ingredients:

- 1 1/2 cups all-purpose flour
- 3/4 cup unsweetened cocoa powder
- 1 teaspoon baking soda
- 1/2 teaspoon baking powder
- 1/4 teaspoon salt
- 1 cup Stevia
- 1/2 cup vegetable oil
- 2 eggs
- 1 cup water

Instructions:

1. Preheat oven to 350 degrees F. Grease and flour one 9x13 inch baking pan.
2. Sift together the flour, cocoa, baking soda, baking powder, and salt. Set aside.
3. In a large bowl, mix together the sugar substitute, oil, eggs, and water. Add the dry ingredients to the wet ingredients and mix until well blended. Pour batter into prepared pan.
4. Bake at 350 degrees F for 30 minutes. Cool cake before serving.

Serving Size: 1 slice
Calories: 250

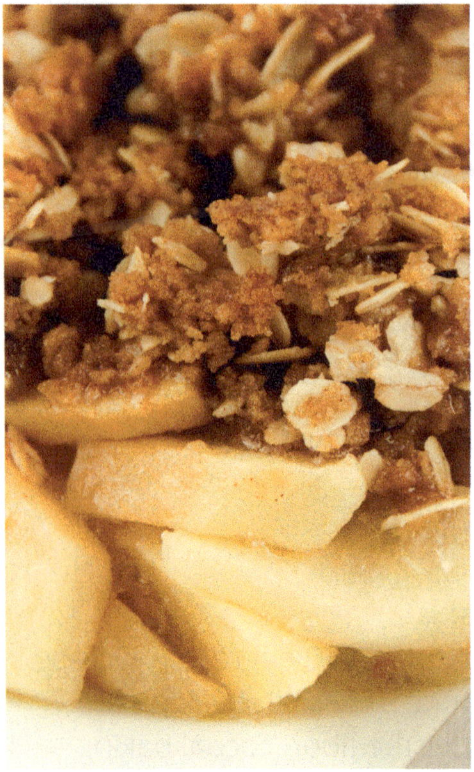

APPLE CRISP

Ingredients:

- 6 large apples, peeled and thinly sliced
- 1/2 cup sugar-free apple juice
- 1/4 cup all-purpose flour
- 1 teaspoon ground cinnamon
- 1/4 teaspoon ground nutmeg

Topping:

- 1/2 cup quick cooking oats
- 1/2 cup brown sugar substitute
- 1/4 cup all-purpose flour
- 1/4 teaspoon baking powder
- 1/4 teaspoon baking soda
- 1/4 teaspoon salt
- 1/4 cup cold butter, cut into small pieces

Instructions:

1. Preheat oven to 375 degrees F.
2. In a large bowl, mix together apples, apple juice, flour, cinnamon, and nutmeg. Pour into a 9x13 inch baking dish.
3. In a medium bowl, mix together oats, brown sugar substitute, flour, baking powder, baking soda, and salt. Cut in butter until mixture resembles coarse crumbs. Sprinkle over the top of the apples.
4. Bake for 30 minutes or until topping is golden brown and apples are tender when pierced with a fork.

Serving Size: 1 piece
Calories: 220

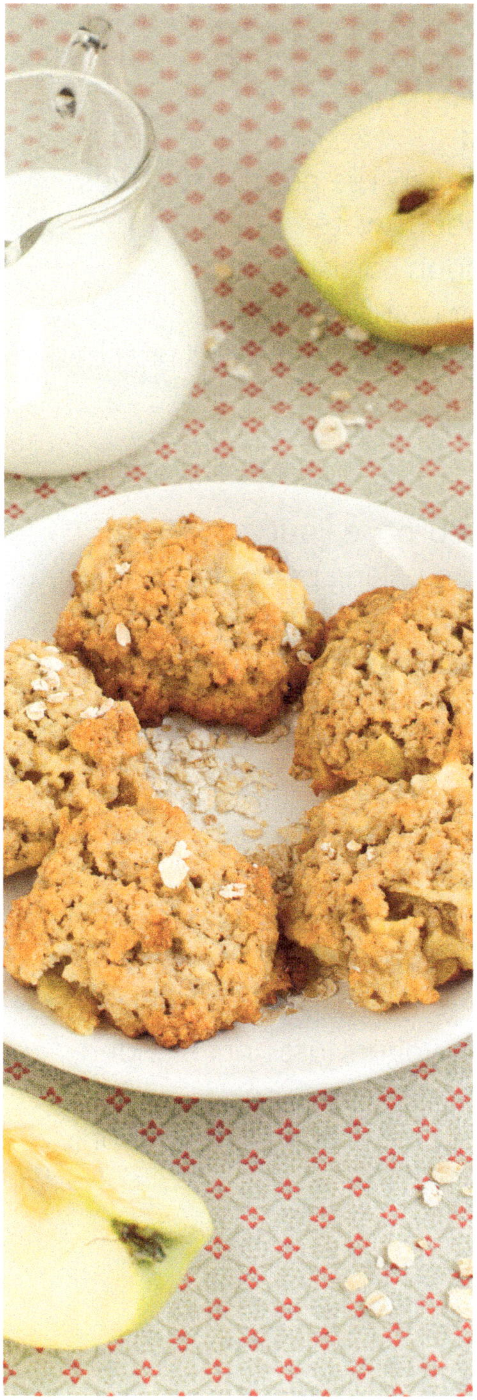

APPLE-OATMEAL COOKIES

Ingredients:

- 1 cup all-purpose flour
- 1 teaspoon baking powder
- 1/2 teaspoon baking soda
- 1/4 teaspoon salt
- 1/2 teaspoon ground cinnamon
- 1/4 teaspoon ground nutmeg
- 1 cup quick cooking oats
- 3/4 cup sugar-free applesauce
- 1 egg, beaten

Instructions:

1. Preheat oven to 375 degrees F. Grease cookie sheets.
2. In a medium bowl, mix together flour, baking powder, baking soda, salt, cinnamon, and nutmeg. Stir in oats. Add applesauce and egg; mix well.
3. Drop dough by rounded tablespoons onto prepared cookie sheets. Bake for 10 minutes or until cookies are lightly browned. Cool on cookie sheets for 5 minutes; remove to wire racks to cool completely.

Serving Size: 1 cookie
Calories: 60

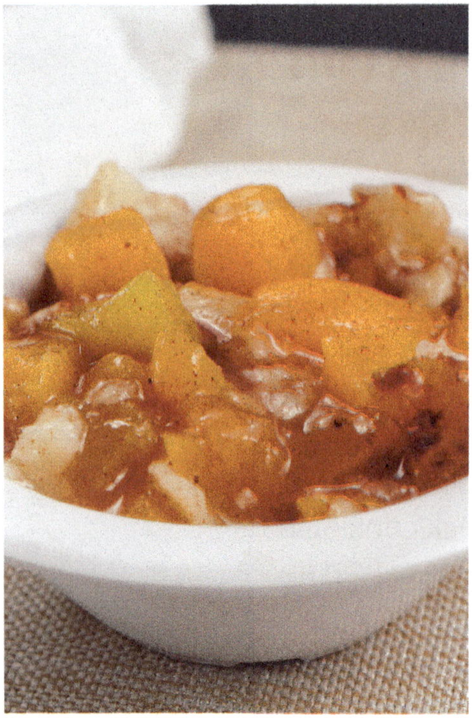

PEACH COBBLER

Ingredients:

- 1/2 cup sugar-free peach preserves
- 2 tablespoons water
- 1 tablespoon cornstarch
- 1 teaspoon vanilla extract
- 4 cups fresh or frozen sliced peaches, thawed and drained

Topping:

- 1 cup all-purpose flour
- 1 teaspoon baking powder
- 1/4 teaspoon salt
- 1/4 cup cold butter, cut into small pieces
- 3/4 cup sugar-free peach yogurt

Instructions:

1. Preheat oven to 375 degrees F. Grease an 8x8 inch baking dish.
2. In a small saucepan, mix together peach preserves, water, cornstarch, and vanilla extract. Cook over low heat until mixture thickens and boils. Remove from heat; stir in peaches. Pour into prepared pan.
3. In a medium bowl, mix together flour, baking powder, and salt. Cut in butter until mixture resembles coarse crumbs. Stir in yogurt just until blended. Drop dough by spoonfuls over the top of the peach mixture.
4. Bake for 25 minutes or until topping is golden brown and filling is bubbly.

Serving Size: 1 piece
Calories: 220

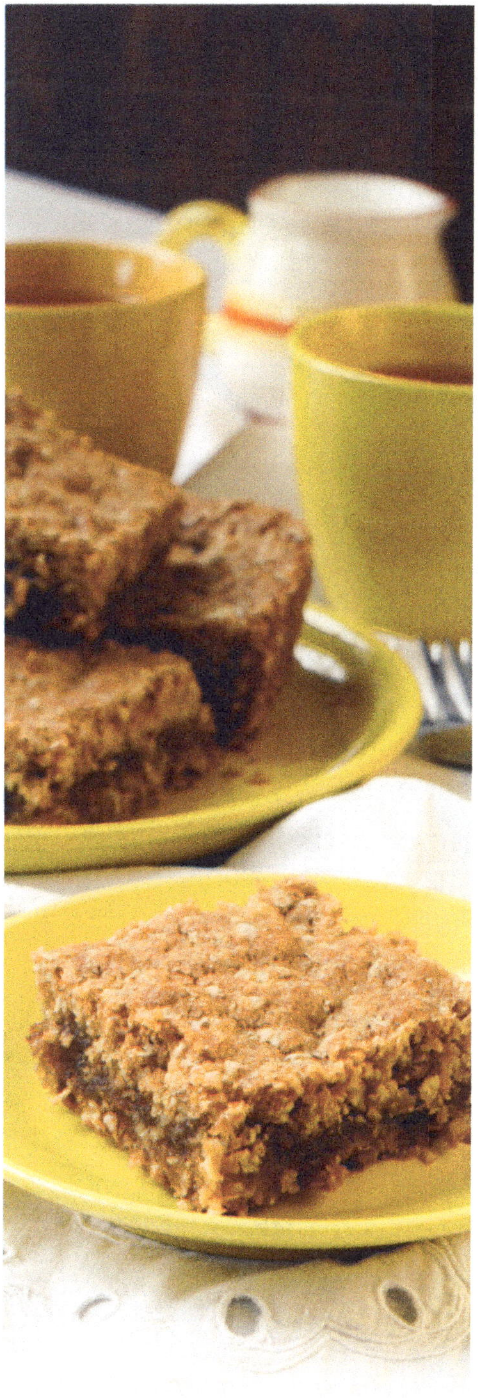

APPLE SQUARES

Ingredients:

- 1/2 cup butter, softened
- 1 cup sugar-free applesauce
- 1 egg, beaten
- 1 teaspoon vanilla extract
- 2 cups all-purpose flour
- 1 teaspoon baking powder
- 1/4 teaspoon baking soda
- 1/4 teaspoon salt

Instructions:

1. Preheat oven to 350 degrees F. Grease and flour an 8x8 inch baking dish.
2. In a large bowl, cream together butter and sugar substitute until light and fluffy. Beat in applesauce, egg, and vanilla extract. In a separate bowl, mix together flour, baking powder, baking soda, and salt. Gradually add to the creamed mixture until well blended. Pour batter into prepared dish.
3. Bake for 25 minutes or until a toothpick inserted into the center comes out clean. Cool in dish on a wire rack. Cut into squares.

Serving Size: 1 square
Calories: 170

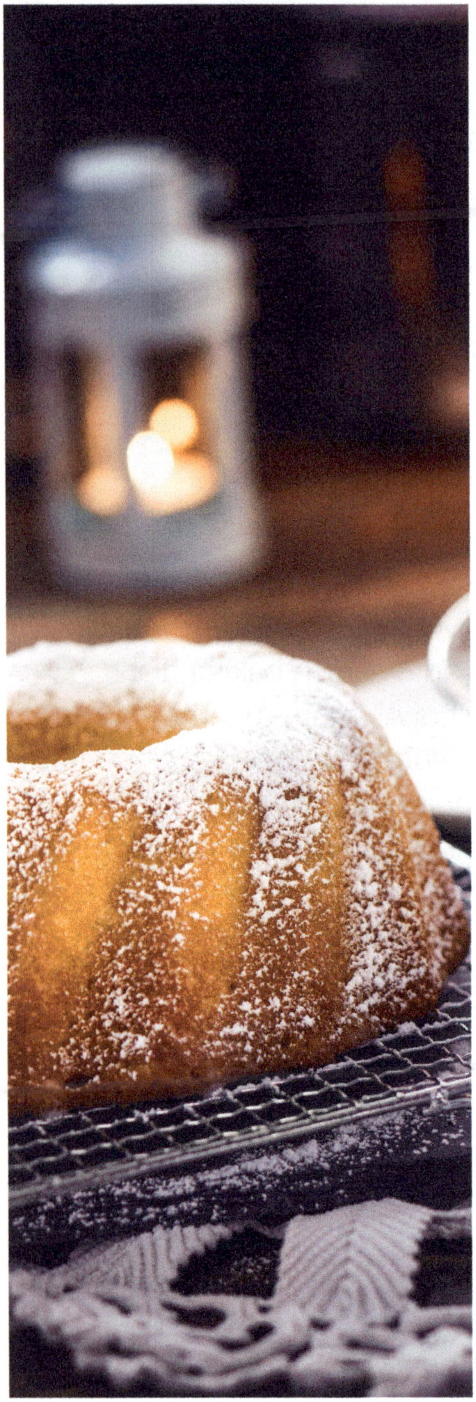

PEAR BUNDT CAKE

Ingredients:

- 1/2 cup butter, softened
- 1 cup sugar-free pear preserves
- 3 eggs
- 1 teaspoon vanilla extract
- 2 cups all-purpose flour
- 1 teaspoon baking powder
- 1/4 teaspoon baking soda
- 1/4 teaspoon salt

Instructions:

1. Preheat oven to 350 degrees F. Grease and flour a bundt cake pan.
2. In a large bowl, cream together butter and sugar substitute until light and fluffy. Beat in pear preserves, eggs, and vanilla extract. In a separate bowl, mix together flour, baking powder, baking soda, and salt. Gradually add to the creamed mixture until well blended. Pour batter into prepared pan.
3. Bake for 45 minutes or until a toothpick inserted into the center comes out clean. Cool in pan on a wire rack for 10 minutes. Remove from pan and cool completely on wire rack.

Serving Size: 1 piece
Calories: 190

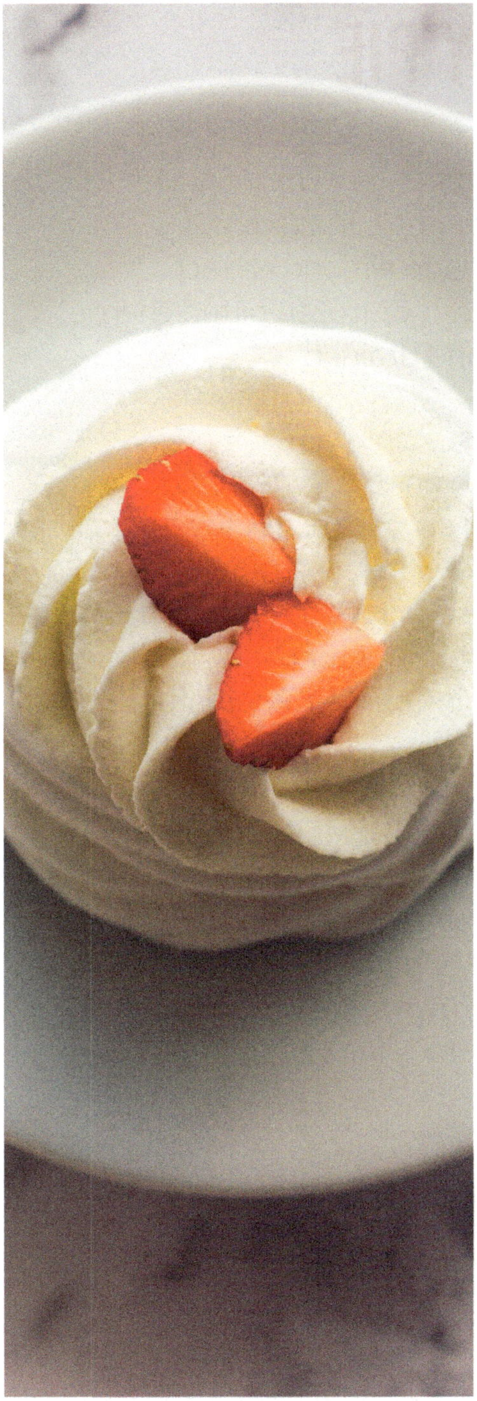

STRAWBERRY PAVLOVA

Ingredients:

- 4 egg whites
- 1/2 teaspoon cream of tartar
- 1 cup sugar-free strawberry preserves

Instructions:

1. Preheat oven to 300 degrees F. Line a baking sheet with parchment paper.
2. In a large bowl, beat egg whites and cream of tartar until foamy. Gradually add sugar substitute, 1 tablespoon at a time, beating constantly until stiff peaks form. Gently fold in strawberry preserves.
3. Drop mixture by spoonful onto prepared baking sheet. Bake for 30 minutes or until meringues are dry and crisp. Cool on baking sheet for 10 minutes; remove to wire racks to cool completely.

Serving Size: 1 meringue
Calories: 60

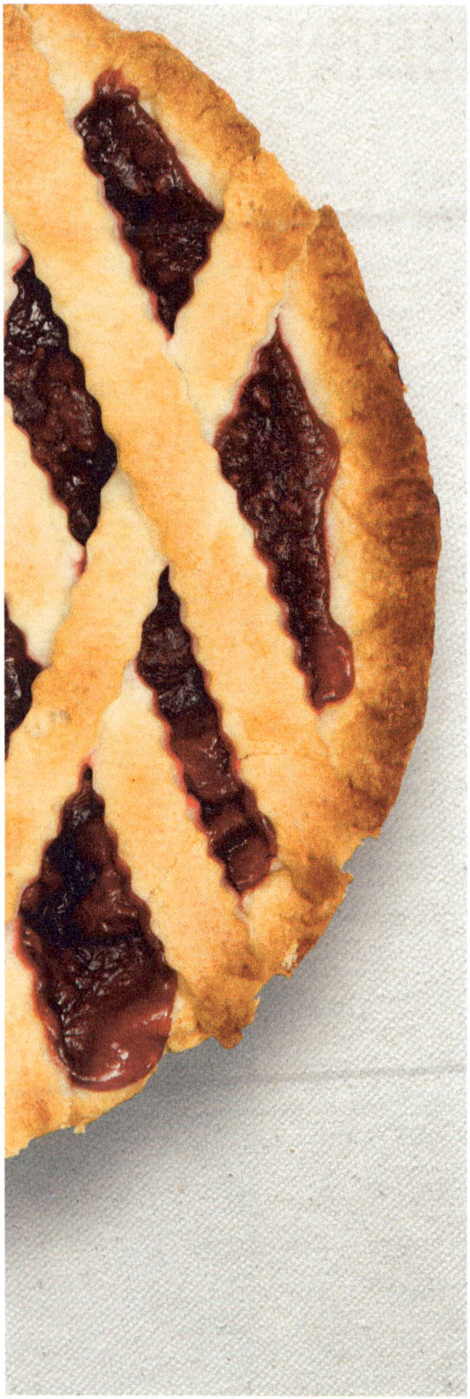

CHERRY PIE

Ingredients:

- 1/2 cup sugar-free cherry preserves
- 2 tablespoons cornstarch
- 1/4 teaspoon almond extract
- 6 cups fresh or frozen pitted cherries, thawed and drained

Instructions:

1. Preheat oven to 375 degrees F.
2. In a small saucepan, mix together cherry preserves, water, cornstarch, and almond extract. Cook over low heat until mixture thickens and boils. Remove from heat; stir in cherries. Pour into an 8 inch pie dish.
3. Cut remaining pastry into 1/2 - 3/4 inch strips. Arrange over top of cherry mixture in a lattice pattern. Trim and flute edges.
4. Bake for 25 minutes or until crust is golden brown and filling is bubbly. Cool on a wire rack for 1 hour before serving.

Serving Size: 1 piece
Calories: 210

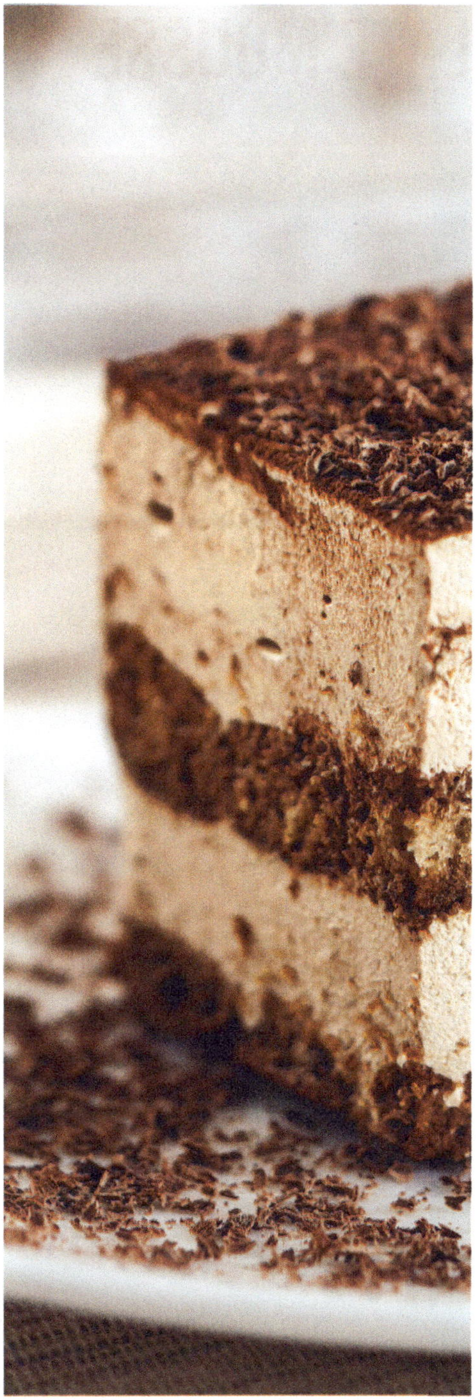

TIRAMISU

Ingredients:

- 1 (16 ounce) package ladyfingers
- 1/2 cup strong brewed coffee, cooled
- 1 (8 ounce) package cream cheese, softened
- 1/4 cup sugar-free vanilla instant pudding mix
- 1 cup cold skim milk
- 1 teaspoon vanilla extract

Instructions:

1. In a small bowl, combine coffee and 1 tablespoon of the sugar substitute. Set aside.
2. In a large bowl, beat cream cheese and remaining sugar substitute until fluffy. Add pudding mix and milk; beat until well blended. Stir in vanilla extract.
3. Split ladyfingers in half lengthwise. Arrange half of the ladyfingers in the bottom of an 8x8 inch dish. Drizzle with half of the coffee mixture. Spread with half of the cream cheese mixture. Repeat layers.
4. Cover and refrigerate for at least 2 hours before serving.

Serving Size: 1 piece
Calories: 210

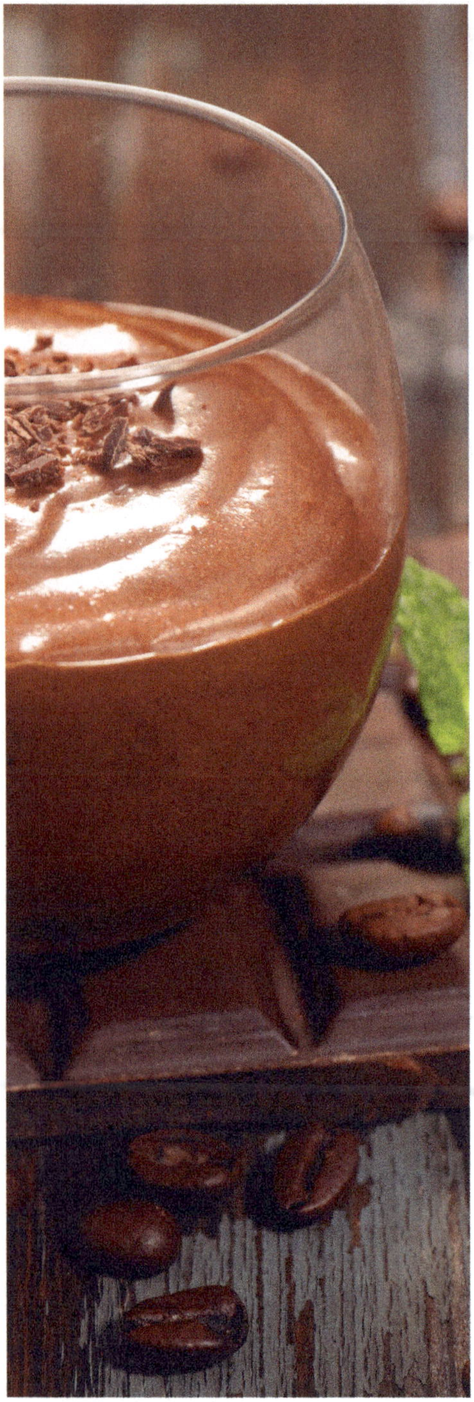

CHOCOLATE MOUSSE

Ingredients:

- 1 (8 ounce) package cream cheese, softened
- 1 cup cold skim milk
- 1/4 cup sugar-free chocolate instant pudding mix

Instructions:

1. In a large bowl, beat cream cheese until fluffy. Add milk and pudding mix; beat until well blended.
2. Pour into individual dishes. Refrigerate for at least 1 hour before serving.

Serving Size: 1 mousse
Calories: 190

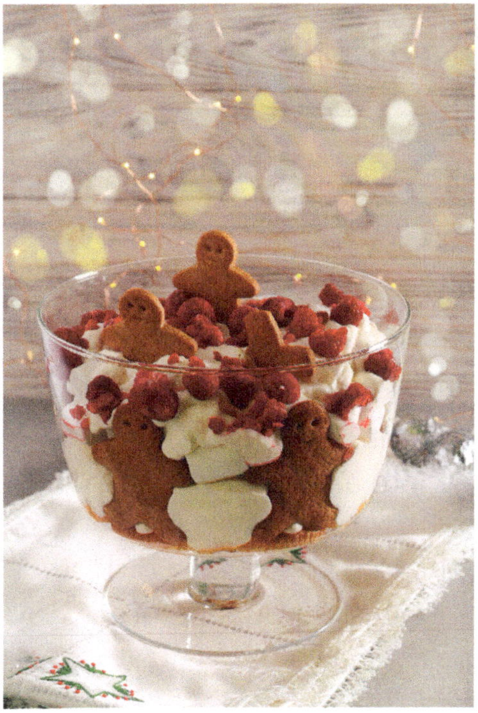

PUMPKIN-BUTTERSCOTCH GINGERBREAD TRIFLE

Ingredients:

- 1 (15 ounce) can pumpkin puree
- 1 cup water
- 3/4 cup sugar-free butterscotch pudding mix
- 1 teaspoon ground ginger
- 1/2 teaspoon ground cinnamon
- 1/4 teaspoon ground cloves
- 1 (12 fluid ounce) container frozen non-dairy whipped topping, thawed

Instructions:

1. In a medium saucepan, mix together pumpkin puree, water, pudding mix, ginger, cinnamon, and cloves. Cook over low heat until mixture thickens and boils. Remove from heat; let cool for 5 minutes.
2. In a large bowl, layer one-third of the pumpkin mixture, one-third of the Gingersnap crumbs, and one-third of the whipped topping. Repeat layers.
3. Cover and refrigerate for at least 2 hours before serving.

Serving Size: 1 trifle
Calories: 420

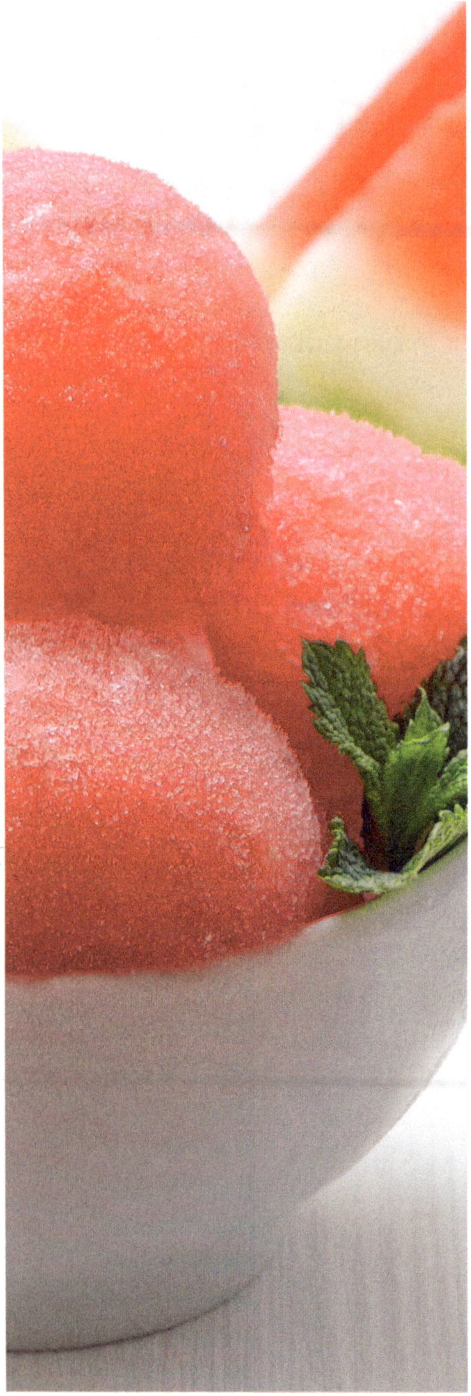

WATERMELON SHERBET

Ingredients:

- 6 cups cubed seedless watermelon
- 1 cup cold skim milk
- 1/2 cup sugar-free strawberry yogurt

Instructions:

1. In a blender or food processor, puree watermelon until smooth.
2. Pour puree into a large bowl; stir in milk and yogurt.
3. Pour mixture into an 8x8 inch dish. Freeze for at least 2 hours before serving.

Serving Size: 1 sherbet
Calories: 90

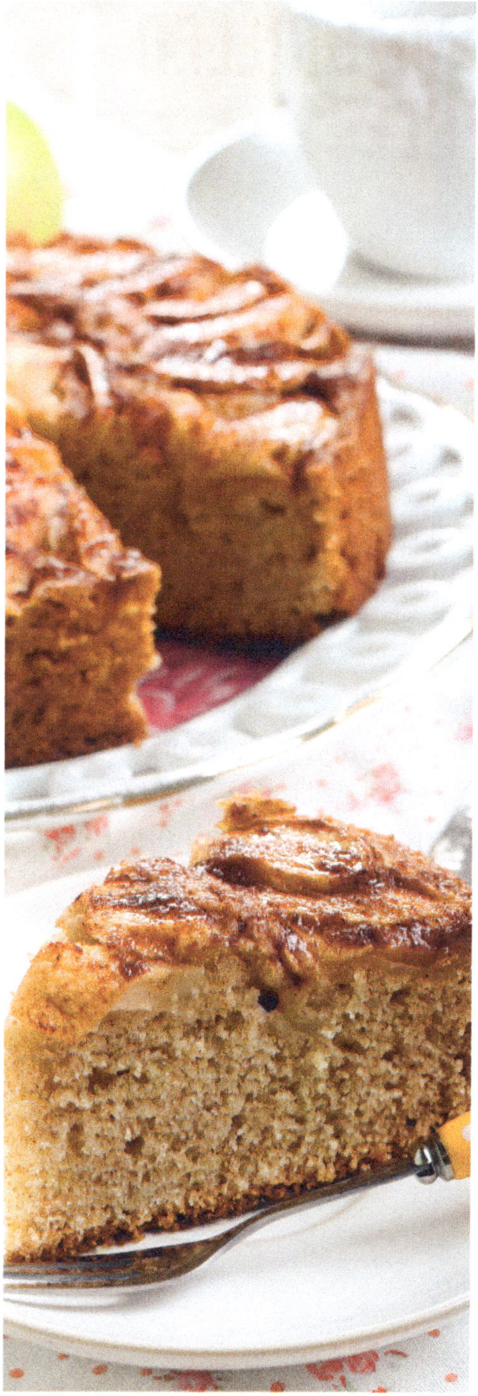

GINGERBREAD TEA CAKE

Ingredients:

- 1 cup cold water
- 1/2 cup sugar-free gingerbread pudding mix

Instructions:

1. Preheat oven to 350 degrees F. Grease and flour an 8x8 inch baking dish.
2. In a medium bowl, whisk together water and pudding mix until well blended. Pour into prepared dish.
3. Bake for 25 minutes or until a toothpick inserted into the center comes out clean. Cool on a wire rack for 5 minutes before serving.

Serving Size: 1 cake
Calories: 170

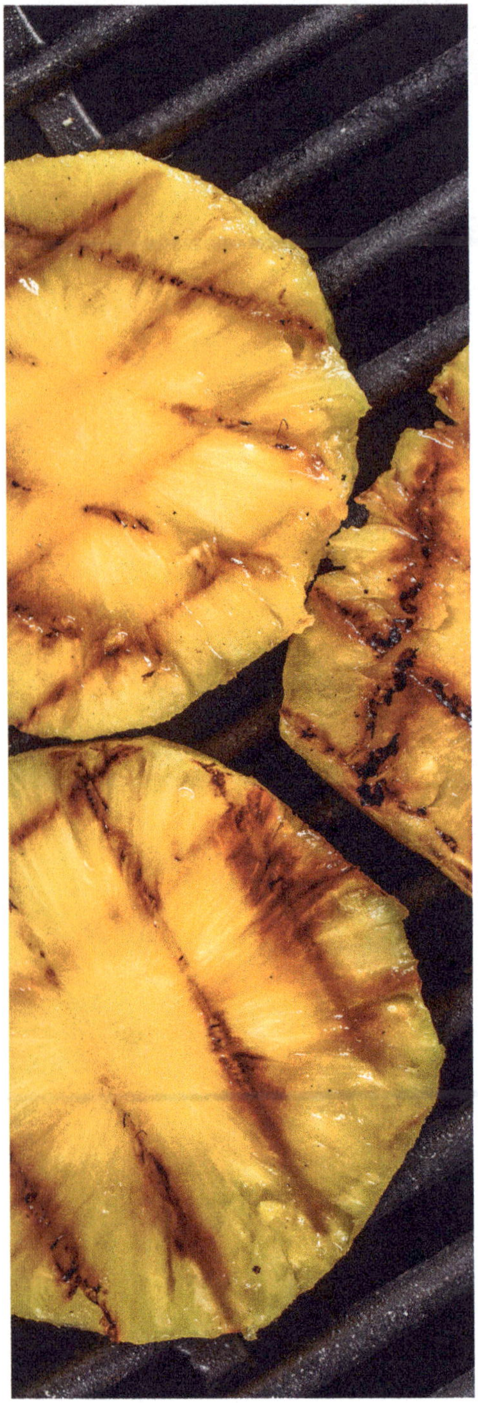

CHILI-LIME GRILLED PINEAPPLE

Ingredients:

- 1 fresh pineapple, peeled, cored, and cut into spears
- 1/4 cup sugar-free limeade concentrate
- 1 tablespoon chili powder

Instructions:

1. Preheat grill to medium-high heat.
2. In a small bowl, whisk together limeade concentrate and chili powder.
3. Grill pineapple spears for 8 minutes or until evenly browned, turning once. Brush with limeade mixture during the last 5 minutes of grilling.
4. Remove from grill; serve immediately.

Serving Size: 1 spear
Calories: 60

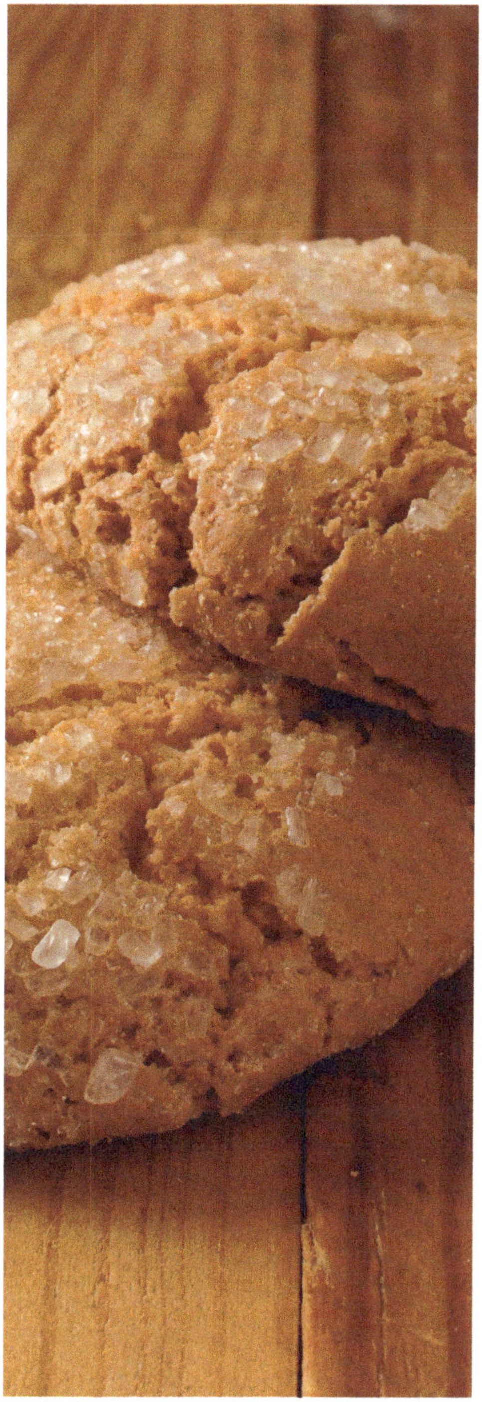

MOLASSES CRACKLE COOKIES

Ingredients:

- 1 cup margarine, softened
- 1 cup sugar-free molasses
- 2 eggs
- 3 cups all-purpose flour
- 2 teaspoons baking soda
- 1 teaspoon ground ginger
- 1/4 teaspoon ground cloves

Instructions:

1. Preheat oven to 350 degrees F. Grease cookie sheets.
2. In a large bowl, cream together margarine and molasses until light and fluffy. Beat in eggs. In a small bowl, whisk together flour, baking soda, ginger, and cloves; gradually add to molasses mixture, mixing until well blended.
3. Drop dough by rounded teaspoons onto prepared cookie sheets. Bake for 10 minutes or until cookies are cracked and set. Cool on wire racks.

Serving Size: 1 cookie
Calories: 140

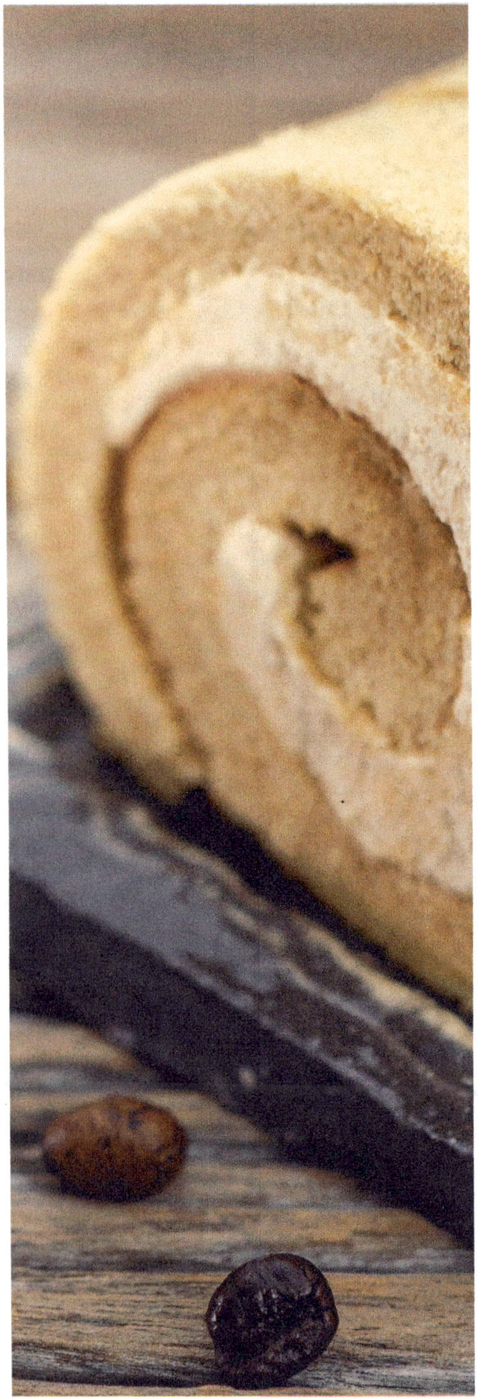

ORANGE RICOTTA CAKE ROLL

Ingredients:

- 1/4 cup margarine, softened
- 1 (15 ounce) container part-skim ricotta cheese
- 3/4 cup sugar-free orange marmalade

Instructions:

1. Preheat oven to 375 degrees F. Grease and flour a 10x15 inch jelly roll pan.
2. In a large bowl, cream together margarine and ricotta cheese until light and fluffy. Stir in orange marmalade. Pour into prepared pan.
3. Bake for 20 minutes or until cake is firm to the touch and golden brown. Cool on a wire rack for 5 minutes; remove from pan and cool completely on wire rack.

Serving Size: 1 slice
Calories: 280

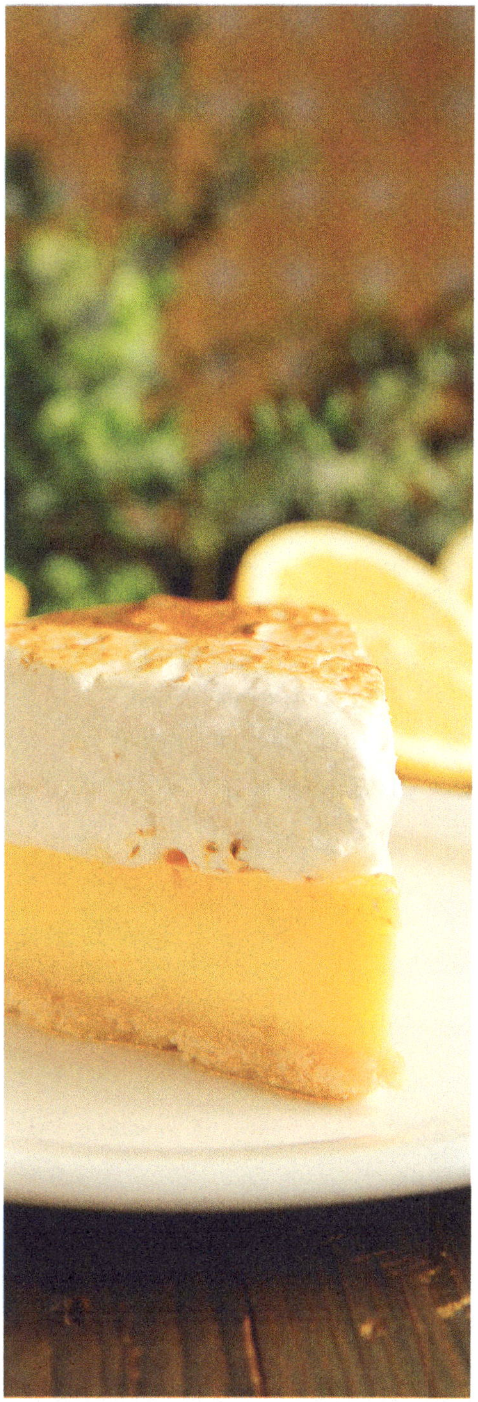

LEMON TOFU CREME PIE

Ingredients:

- 1 (14 ounce) package extra firm tofu, drained
- 1/2 cup sugar-free lemonade concentrate

Instructions:

1. Preheat oven to 350 degrees F. Grease a 9 inch pie dish.
2. In a food processor or blender, puree tofu until smooth. Add lemonade concentrate and blend until well combined. Pour into prepared dish.
3. Bake for 25 minutes or until firm to the touch and slightly golden brown. Cool on a wire rack for 5 minutes before serving.

Serving Size: 1 slice
Calories: 190

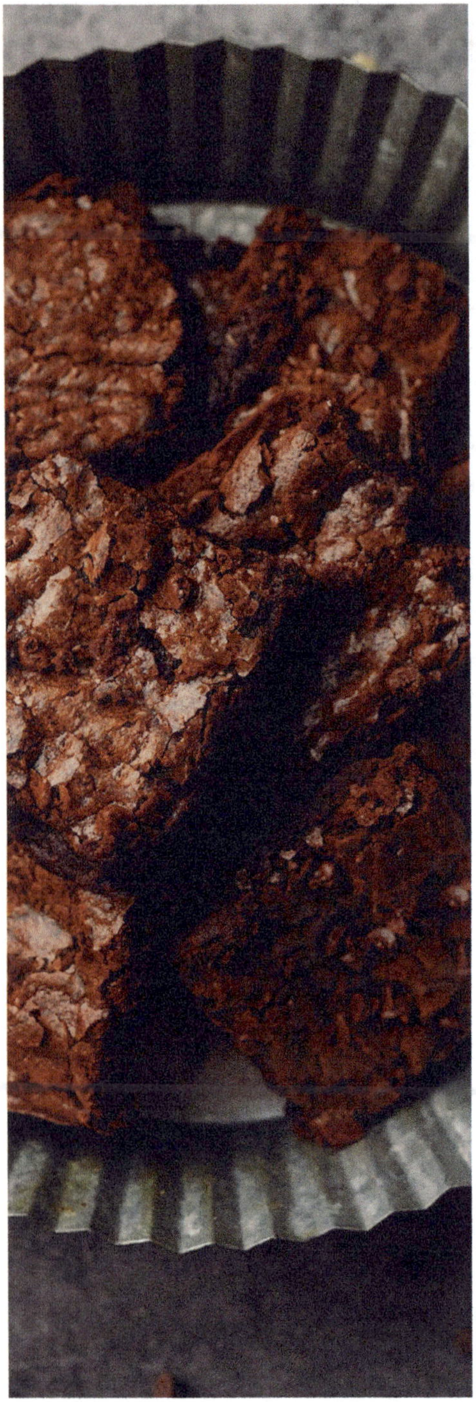

RASPBERRY COCOA SQUARES

Ingredients:

- 1/4 cup margarine, melted
- 1 cup all-purpose flour
- 1 cup sugar-free raspberry jam

Instructions:

1. Preheat oven to 350 degrees F. Grease an 8x8 inch baking dish.
2. In a medium bowl, whisk together margarine and flour until well blended; press into the bottom of prepared dish. Spread raspberry jam over crust.
3. Bake for 25 minutes or until golden brown. Cool on a wire rack for 5 minutes before serving.

Serving Size: 1 square
Calories: 210

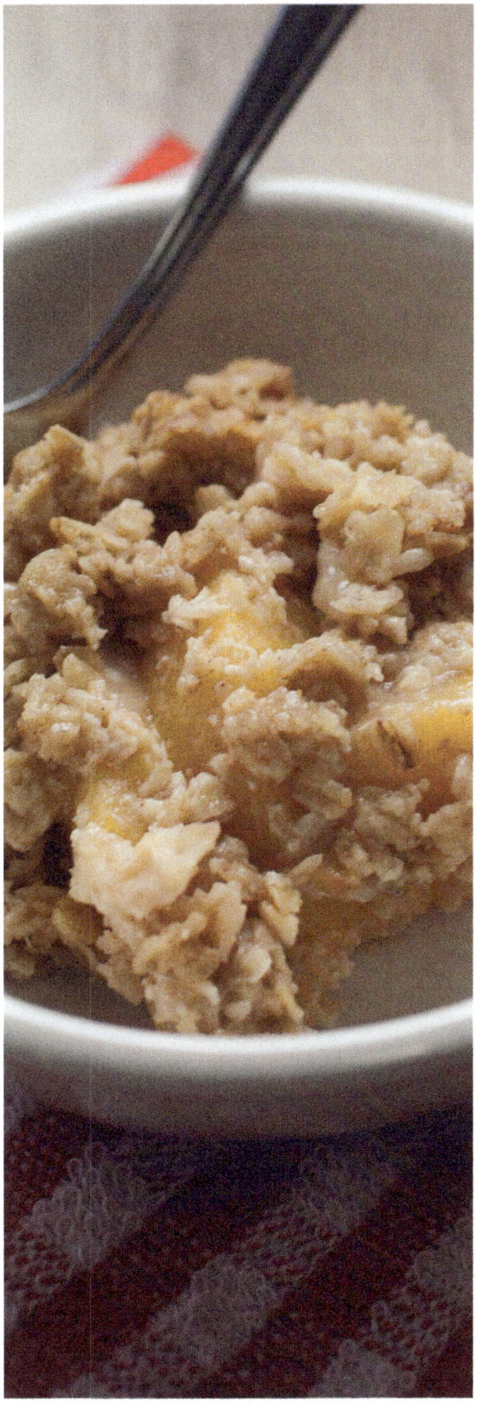

PEACH CRISP

Ingredients:

- 4 cups sliced fresh peaches
- 1/4 cup sugar-free peach preserves

Instructions:

1. Preheat oven to 375 degrees F. Grease a 9 inch baking dish.
2. In a large bowl, mix together peaches and peach preserves. Pour into prepared dish.
3. Bake for 20 minutes or until bubbly and peaches are tender. Cool on a wire rack for 5 minutes before serving.

Serving Size: 1/2 cup
Calories: 120

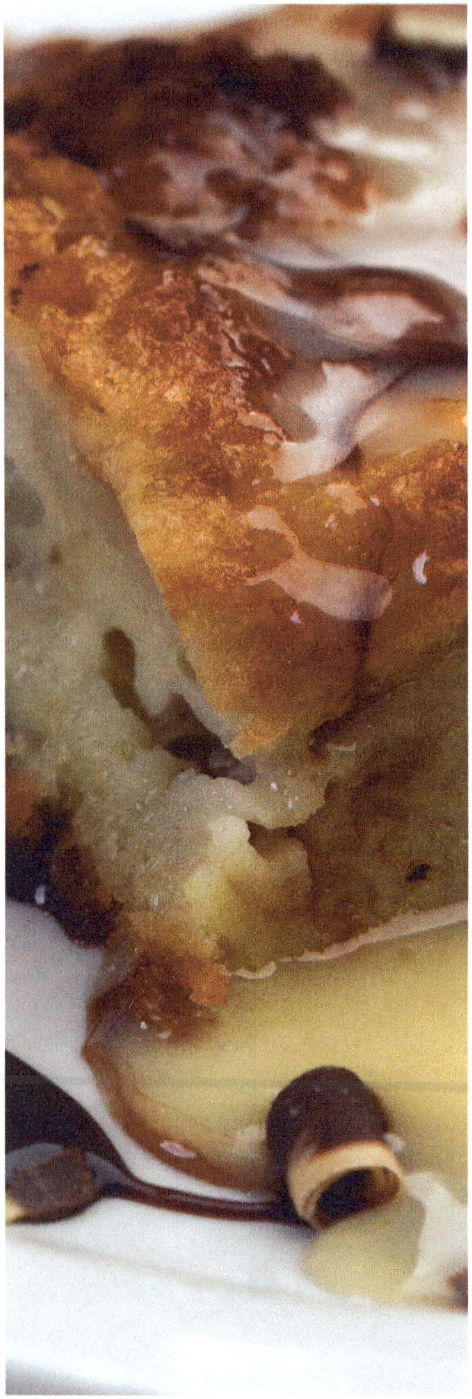

BANANA NUT BREAD PUDDING

Ingredients:

- 1 (16 ounce) loaf sugar-free banana nut bread, cubed
- 1 cup skim milk
- 3 eggs, beaten

Instructions:

1. Preheat oven to 350 degrees F. Grease a 9x13 inch baking dish.
2. In a large bowl, mix together banana bread cubes, milk, and eggs. Pour into prepared dish.
3. Bake for 30 minutes or until pudding is set. Cool on a wire rack for 5 minutes before serving.

Serving Size: 1/2 cup
Calories: 190

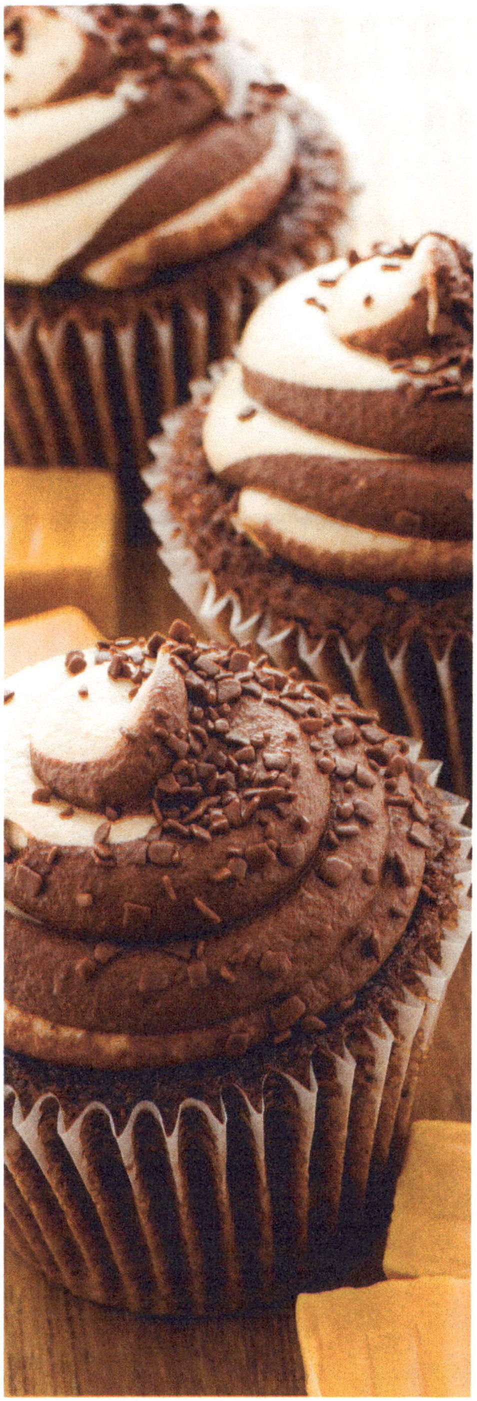

CHOCOLATE MACAROON CUPCAKES

Ingredients:

- 1/2 cup margarine, softened
- 3/4 cup sugar-free chocolate syrup
- 2 eggs
- 1 teaspoon vanilla extract
- 1 1/2 cups all-purpose flour

Instructions:

1. Preheat oven to 350 degrees F. Grease 24 muffin cups.
2. In a large bowl, cream together margarine and chocolate syrup until light and fluffy. Beat in eggs one at a time, then stir in vanilla extract. In a small bowl, whisk together flour and baking soda; gradually add to chocolate mixture, mixing just until blended.
3. Fill prepared muffin cups three-quarters full with batter. Bake for 15 minutes or until a toothpick inserted into the center of a cupcake comes out clean. Cool on a wire rack for 5 minutes; remove from pan and cool completely on wire rack.

Serving Size: 1 cupcake
Calories: 210

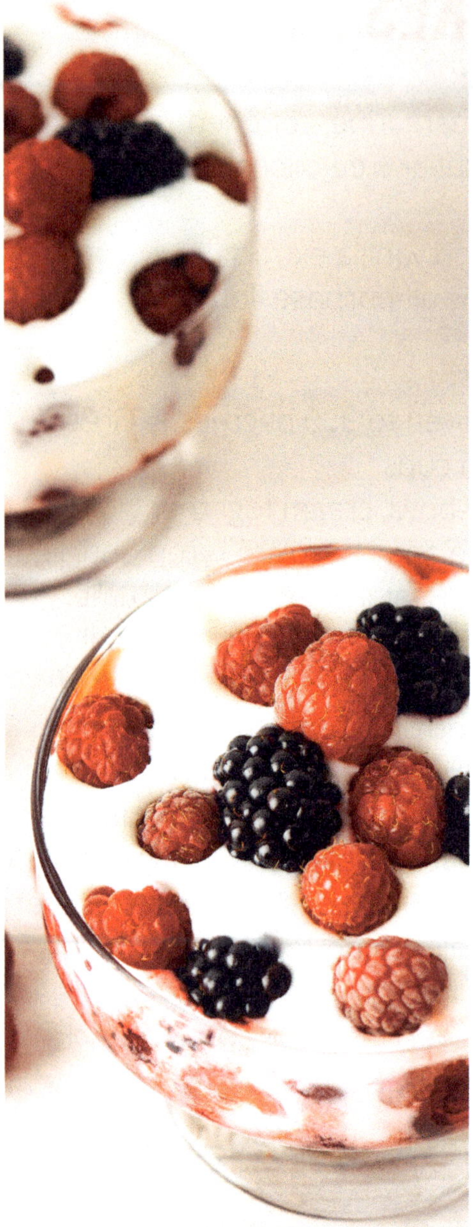

SOUR CREAM BAVARIAN

Ingredients:

- 1 quart sour cream
- 1 (3 ounce) package sugar-free raspberry gelatin mix

Instructions:

1. In a medium bowl, whisk together sour cream and raspberry gelatin mix until well blended. Pour into a 9x13 inch dish.
2. Refrigerate for 4 hours or until firm. Cut into squares and serve.

Serving Size: 1 square
Calories: 90

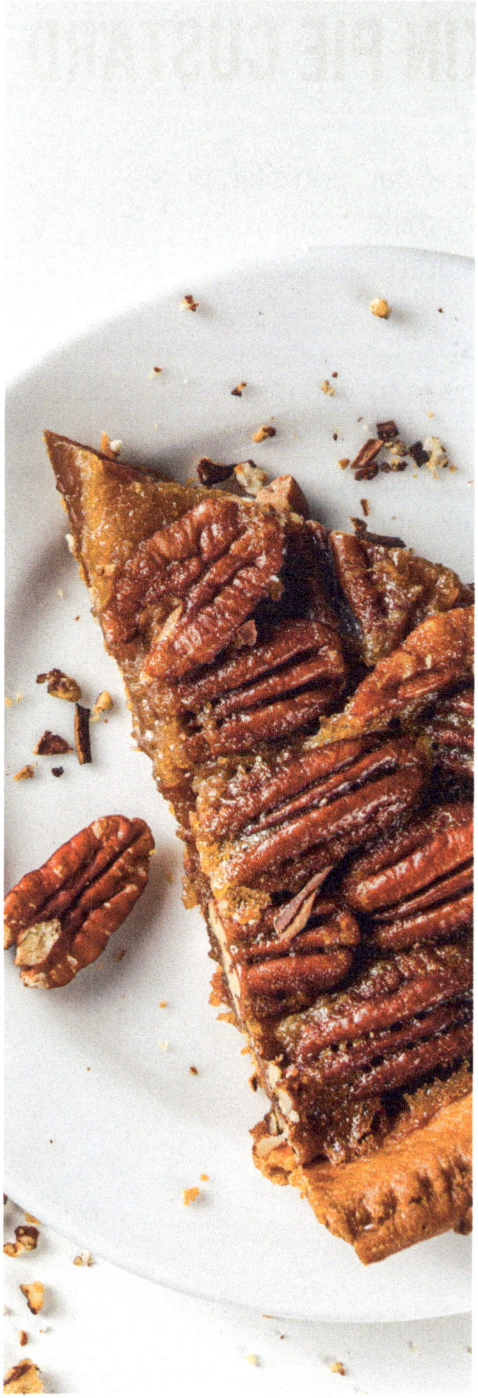

MAPLE PECAN PIE

Ingredients:

- 1 unbaked 9 inch pie crust
- 1 cup chopped pecans
- 3 eggs, beaten
- 1 cup sugar-free syrup

Instructions:

1. Preheat oven to 350 degrees F.
2. In a medium bowl, mix together pecans, eggs, and syrup. Pour into pie crust.
3. Bake for 40 minutes or until pie is set and crust is golden brown. Cool on a wire rack for 5 minutes before serving.

Serving Size: 1 slice
Calories: 280

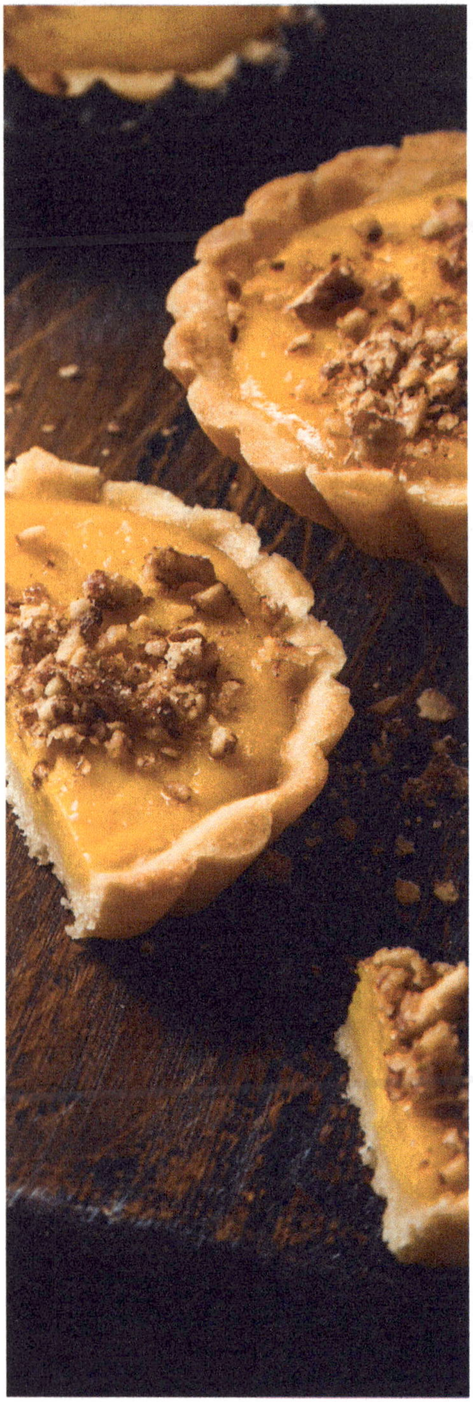

PUMPKIN PIE CUSTARD

Ingredients:

- 1 (15 ounce) can pumpkin puree
- 1 cup skim milk
- 3 eggs, beaten

Instructions:

1. Preheat oven to 350 degrees F. Grease a 9x13 inch baking dish.
2. In a large bowl, whisk together pumpkin puree, milk, and eggs. Pour into prepared dish.
3. Bake for 40 minutes or until custard is set. Cool on a wire rack for 5 minutes before serving.

Serving Size: 1/2 cup
Calories: 80

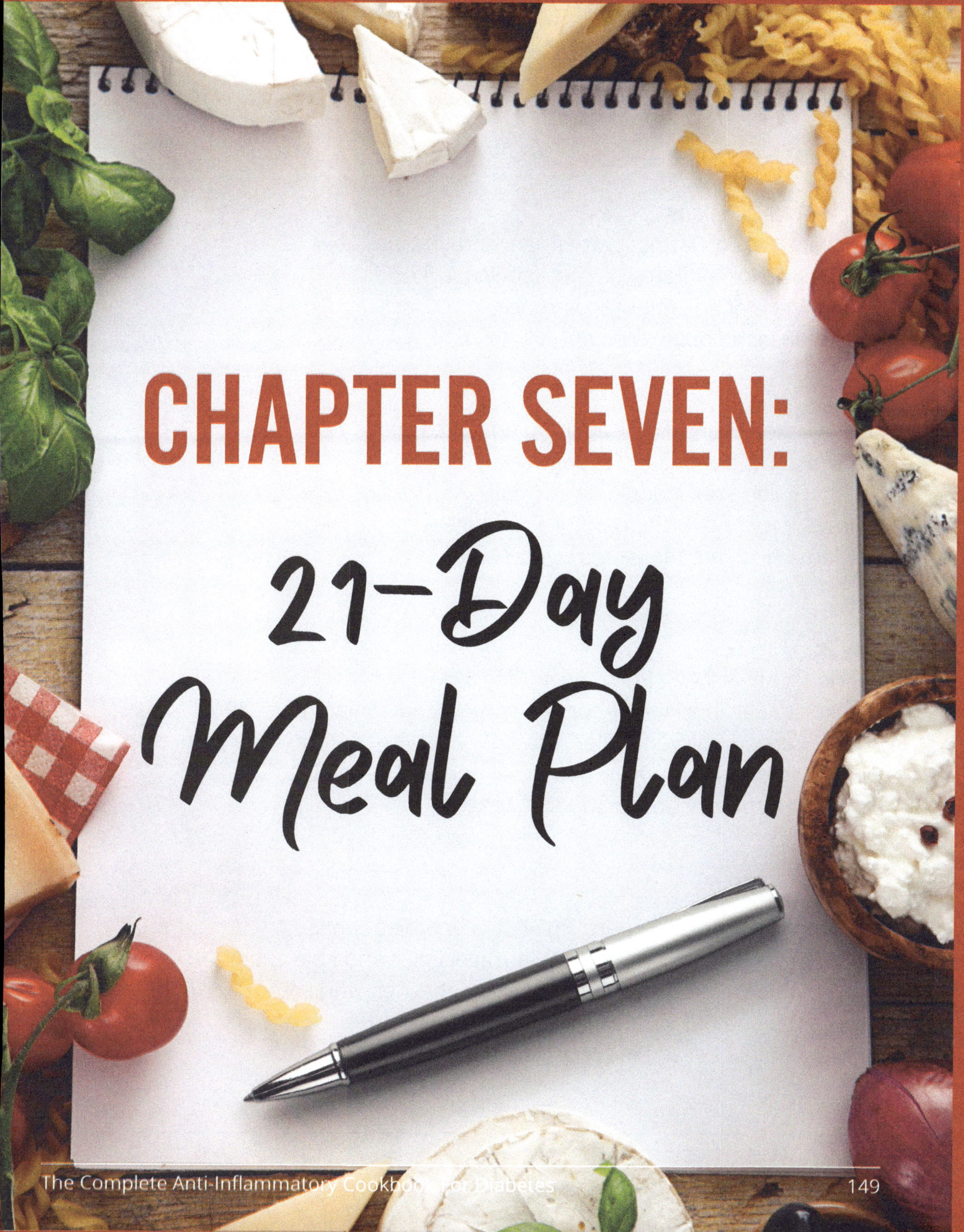

CHAPTER SEVEN:

21-Day Meal Plan

21-DAY MEAL PLAN

Day 1:
Snack: Spiced Pecans *..page 7*
Breakfast: Baked Oatmeal with Pears and Pecans *..page 32*
Lunch: Artichoke Ratatouille Chicken *..page 83*
Dinner: Vegetarian Lentil Tacos *..page 90*
Dessert: Peach Cobbler *..page 128*

Day 2:
Snack: Baked Broccoli-Cheddar Quinoa Bites *..page 12*
Breakfast: Omelet in a Mug *..page 38*
Lunch: Grilled Pork Noodle Salad *..page 77*
Dinner: Spicy Beef & Pepper Stir-Fry *..page 98*
Dessert: Chocolate Mousse *..page 134*

Day 3:
Snack: Southwest Egg Rolls *..page 18*
Breakfast: "Egg in a Hole" Peppers with Avocado Salsa *..page 39*
Lunch: Curried Chicken Skillet *..page 69*
Dinner: Ginger-Tahini Oven-Baked Salmon and Vegetables *..page 93*
Dessert: Raspberry Cocoa Squares *..page 142*

Day 4:
Snack: Cucumber Dill Yogurt Dip with Vegetables *..page 24*
Breakfast: Cauliflower Hash with Sausage, Eggs, and Kale *..page 44*
Lunch: Quinoa Salad with Edamame, Cranberries, and Feta *..page 66*
Dinner: Quinoa Black Bean Burrito Bowl *..page 103*
Dessert: Maple Pecan Pie *..page 147*

Day 5:

Snack: Jalapeno Poppers *..page 25*

Breakfast: Tomato-Parmesan Mini Quiches *..page 49*

Lunch: Cucumber, Avocado, and Rice Sushi Rolls *..page 67*

Dinner: Spinach Rolls *..page 116*

Dessert: Chocolate Macaroon Cupcakes *..page 145*

Day 6:

Snack: Air Fryer Plantain Chips *..page 2*

Breakfast: Salmon Cucumber Roll-Ups *..page 52*

Lunch: Chicken with Fire-Roasted Tomatoes and Quinoa *..page 74*

Dinner: Cod with Hearty Tomato Sauce *..page 122*

Dessert: Lemon Tofu Creme Pie *..page 141*

Day 7:

Snack: Cheesy Kale Chips *..page 4*

Breakfast: Meyer Lemon Avocado Toast *..page 33*

Lunch: Simple Sesame Chicken with Couscous *..page 80*

Dinner: Meaty Slow-Cooked Jambalaya *..page 117*

Dessert: Watermelon Sherbet *..page 136*

Day 8:

Snack: Baked Sweet Potato Coins *..page 8*

Breakfast: Spinach and Egg Scramble with Raspberries on Toast *..page 29*

Lunch: Turkey Chili with Sweet Potatoes *..page 75*

Dinner: Chicken Taco Salad with Cilantro Lime Dressing *..page 108*

Dessert: Cherry Pie *..page 132*

Day 9:

Snack: Spicy Roasted Chickpeas ..*page 3*
Breakfast: Curried Chicken Salad Lettuce Wraps ..*page 53*
Lunch: Thin-Crust Vegetable Pizza ..*page 65*
Dinner: Banh Mi Chicken Burger Lettuce Wraps ..page *102*
Dessert: Apple-Oatmeal Cookies ..page *127*

Day 10:

Snack: Garlic White Bean Dip with Celery Sticks ..*page 11*
Breakfast: Peanut Butter and Fig Roasted Flatbread ..*page 51*
Lunch: Sweet Pepper-Green Onion Quesadillas ..*page 60*
Dinner: Spicy Sausage and Potato Soup ..*page 95*
Dessert: Ginger Plum Tart ..*page 124*

Day 11:

Snack: Asian Wraps ..*page 19*
Breakfast: Apple Crisp Oatmeal Bowl ..*page 45*
Lunch: Turkey Avocado BLT Sandwich on Whole Wheat Bread ..*page 56*
Dinner: Roasted Salmon with Asparagus and Potatoes ..*page 87*
Dessert: Chocolate Cake ..*page 125*

Day 12:

Snack: Balsamic-Goat Cheese Grilled Plums ..*page 16*
Breakfast: Banana Peanut Butter Breakfast Smoothie ..*page 42*
Lunch: Greek Yogurt Chicken Salad Wrap with Grapes ..*page 55*
Dinner: Chicken and Spinach Skillet Pasta with Lemon and Garlic ..*page 85*
Dessert: Pear Bundt Cake ..*page 130*

Day 13:

Snack: Roasted Red Pepper Tapenade ..*page 23*
Breakfast: Turkey, Apple, and Cheddar Sandwich ..*page 43*
Lunch: Whole-Grain Pasta With Turkey and Veggies ..*page 62*
Dinner: Cream of Turkey and Wild Rice Soup ..*page 92*
Dessert: Pumpkin-Butterscotch Gingerbread Trifle ..*page 135*

Day 14:

Snack: Frozen Yogurt-Covered Strawberries *..page 17*
Breakfast: Savory Oatmeal with Bananas, almonds, & strawberries *..page 40*
Lunch: Egg Salad Sandwich on Whole Wheat Bread *..page 58*
Dinner: Creamy Fettuccine with Brussels Sprouts and Mushrooms *..page 99*
Dessert: Orange Ricotta Cake Roll *..page 140*

Day 15:

Snack: Basil and Pesto Hummus with Pita Chips *..page 13*
Breakfast: Spinach Egg White Muffins *..page 48*
Lunch: Tuna Teriyaki Kabobs with Brown Rice *..page 72*
Dinner: Skinny Chicken Enchiladas *..page 106*
Dessert: Banana Nut Bread Pudding *..page 144*

Day 16:

Snack: Savory Date and Pistachio Bites *..page 9*
Breakfast: Breakfast Salad with Soft-Boiled Eggs and Salsa Verde Vinaigrette *..page 50*
Lunch: Salmon with Mango Salsa *..page 79*
Dinner: Grilled Beef Chimichangas with Pico de Gallo *..page 104*
Dessert: Sour Cream Bavarian *..page 146*

Day 17:

Snack: Roasted Cauliflower with Tahini Sauce *..page 10*
Breakfast: Greek Yogurt Pancakes *..page 37*
Lunch: Fish Tacos with Berry Salsa *..page 73*
Dinner: Healthy Slow Cooker Chicken Tikka Masala *..page 96*
Dessert: Pumpkin Pie Custard *..page 148*

Day 18:
Snack: Apricot-Ginger Energy Balls *..page 15*
Breakfast: Bean and Bacon Breakfast Tacos *..page 34*
Lunch: Lemon Shrimp and Orzo Salad *..page 68*
Dinner: Tropical Chicken Cauliflower Rice Bowls *..page 91*
Dessert: Chili-Lime Grilled Pineapple *..page 138*

Day 19:
Snack: Cinnamon Roasted Almonds *..page 6*
Breakfast: Pumpkin Spice Oatmeal with Dried Cranberries *..page 31*
Lunch: Stuffed Sweet Potatoes with Salsa and Beans *..page 64*
Dinner: Slow-Cooker Braised Beef with Carrots and Turnips *..page 88*
Dessert: Gingerbread Tea Cake *..page 137*

Day 20:
Snack: Blueberry Lemon Energy Balls *..page 5*
Breakfast: Sausage, Egg, and Cheese Breakfast Casserole *..page 35*
Lunch: Egg and Broccoli Slaw Wrap with Tzatziki Sauce *..page 63*
Dinner: Skillet Pork Chops with Apples and Onion *..page 101*
Dessert: Tiramisu *..page 133*

Day 21:
Snack: Strawberry-Chocolate Greek Yogurt Bark *..page 14*
Breakfast: Ham and Cheese Breakfast Sliders *..page 36*
Lunch: Salmon Poke Bowl with Brown Rice *..page 61*
Dinner: Beef and Rice Stuffed Cabbage Rolls *..page 114*
Dessert: Molasses Crackle Cookies *..page 139*

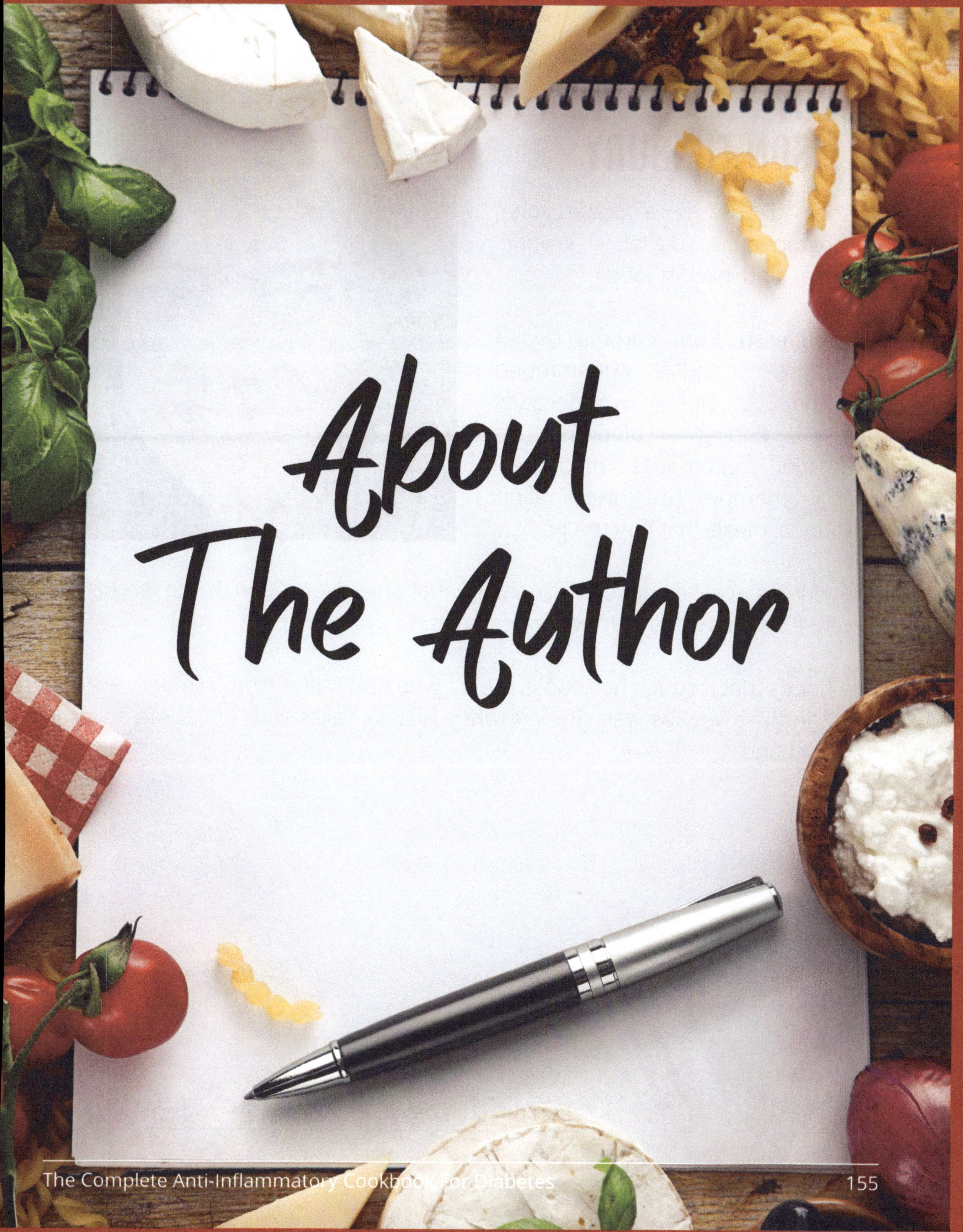

About The Author

ABOUT ALLISON TUXBURY

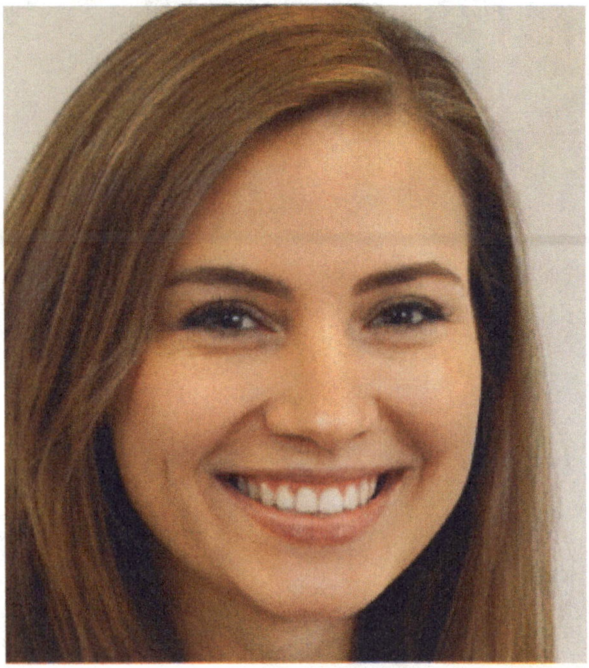

Allison Tuxbury is a professional photographer, digital graphic designer, and lover of food.

She suffered from chronic health conditions and autoimmune symptoms for nearly two decades before finding solutions in meditation, alternative medicines, energy therapy, breathwork, and nutritional meals that fuel the body.

She writes because she loves to share what she's learned with the world, and because it's fun to come up with new meals.

She hopes that through her books others who also suffer from ailments will find relief and recovery as well. She currently lives in Texas with her three children and husband.

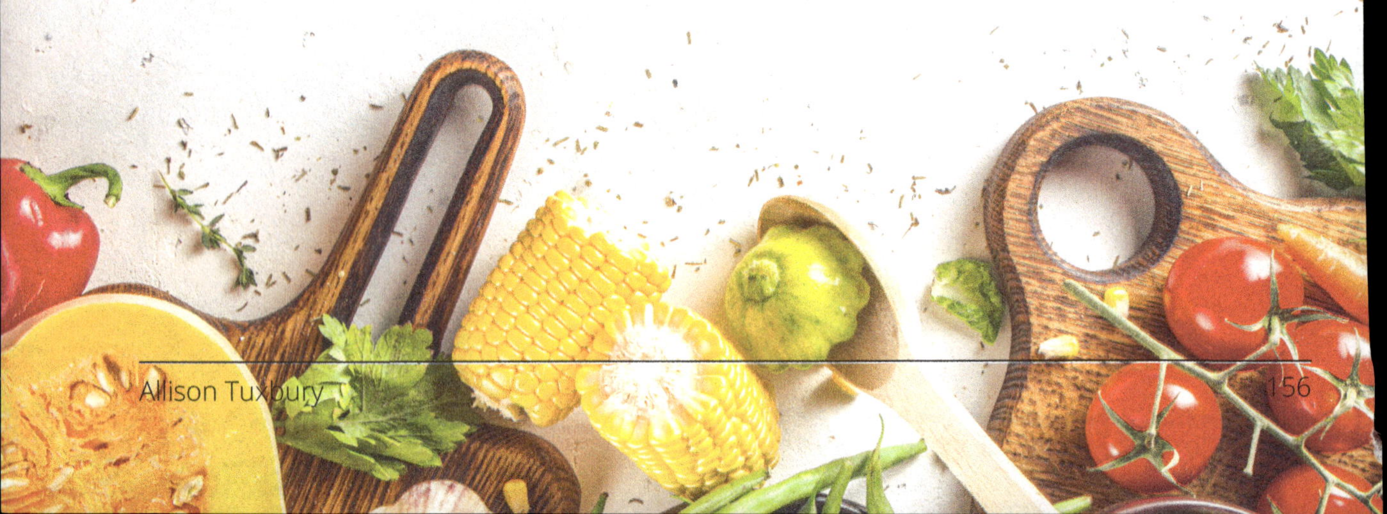

INDEX

INDEX

INDEX

INDEX

Copyright © 2022 Allison Tuxbury
All rights reserved. No part of this guide may be reproduced in any form without permission in writing from the publisher except in the case of brief quotations embodied in critical articles or reviews.

Made in the USA
Monee, IL
09 February 2023

27124835R00103